STARVING
FOR
SURVIVAL

ONE MAN'S JOURNEY WITH ORTHOREXIA

STARVING

FOR

SURVIVAL

ONE MAN'S JOURNEY WITH ORTHOREXIA

JASON WOOD

FOREWORD BY DR. JASON NAGATA

Starving for Survival: One Man's Journey With Orthorexia by Jason Wood
Orthorexia Bites, LLC

Copyright 2022 by Jason Wood

For more information or to book an author event, contact Jason Wood at jason@orthorexiabites.com or visit the website at orthorexiabites.com.

PUBLISHED BY
Orthorexia Bites
Orthorexiabites.com
jason@orthorexiabites.com
Denver, Colorado

ISBN: 978-1-7379231-0-7 (paperback)
          978-1-7379231-1-4 (epub)

CONTENTS

FOREWORD

Early in my medical training, I developed an interest in caring for young people with eating disorders, particularly boys and men. After witnessing delays in diagnosis, challenges with receiving appropriate treatment, and stigmatization with this female-centric disease, I dedicated my career to research and clinical care for boys and men with eating disorders. I recently edited the book *Eating Disorders in Boys and Men* to provide up-to-date guidance for clinicians on the topic.

Eating disorders in men are underrecognized, largely because men's stories with body image and eating disorders remain untold. I first heard Jason Wood's story through his outspoken advocacy on the subject. He has bravely shared his own experiences with an eating disorder through his website, blog posts, podcasts, and interviews.

Jason's memoir, *Starving for Survival,* is a vivid page-turner that depicts his journey with an eating disorder from his childhood through adult life. He bravely shares his innermost thoughts, vulnerabilities, and experiences, which can be intensely personal and challenging. It is rare to read such introspection coupled with details into the thought process of someone's innermost battles with an eating disorder. Throughout Jason's story, I admire his resilience through the many challenges life sent his way. I couldn't help but root for him as he faced childhood adversity, fell in love, and confronted his illness. It was educational for me as a physician to hear his full life story from childhood and how family illness, bullying, conflict, poverty, and substance abuse shaped his life.

Jason's story highlighted for me some important lessons supported by research regarding eating disorders in men. First, adverse childhood experiences, bullying, and teasing can have a lasting impact on children's mental and physical health. Taunts of "Fatty" and "Porkchop" in the middle school locker room clearly left a lasting impression on Jason's self-esteem and image for decades to come. Jason's story is a reminder of the importance of addressing these issues early on as a pediatrician.

Eating disorders can affect people of all sizes, and people with higher weights actually experience the highest rates of disordered eating behaviors to lose weight. Eating disorders can present in unique ways especially in men, and Jason's path was through a well-meaning pursuit of "clean" and "healthy" eating, which evolved into an obsession and preoccupation with healthy eating, known as orthorexia. Furthermore, the COVID-19 pandemic, which increased social isolation, anxiety related to the pandemic, and disruptions in normal routines, has led to a surge in eating disorder symptoms and referrals. Jason's story highlights how the pandemic precipitated a relapse along the road to recovery.

Starving for Survival served as a call for me to double down on efforts to raise awareness, continue research, develop new treatments, and advocate for more services for men with eating disorders. Health care providers need more training in identifying eating disorders in men and other diverse populations so that we can better support people like Jason through their challenges. I hope that Jason's story will be an important step in inspiring others to share their stories, combat stigma, and help to recognize signs and symptoms of eating disorders. I hope you will learn much from his courageous story.

Jason M. Nagata, MD, MSc
Department of Pediatrics
University of California, San Francisco

CHAPTER 1

REFUGE LOST

My dad swore McDonald's had healing powers. From our spots in a booth next to the door, we watched his hypothesis play out each day after school. Hungry customers, heads down, walked past the images of Ronald McDonald and Grimace. A few minutes later, we watched these same families and couples walk out, grinning ear to ear with a happy meal in hand. Lo and behold, the old man was on to something.

I can attest to the buzz. Well, at least from a five-year-old's perspective. My biggest concern was wondering which Changeables toy I'd get in the Happy Meal box, like my favorite, the fry box that morphed into a dinosaur.

My burgers had to be plain, except for pickles. The tangy crunch paired perfectly with the steamed bun and chewy beef patty. After a bite into the burger, I'd dip the nuggets and French fries into the small plastic container of smokey barbeque sauce. It was a sad day when they discontinued the supersize order of those crispy, salty fries. A large never felt like enough.

To finish off the meal, I'd order soft-serve ice cream cones and apple pies, even though the gooey filling burnt the roof of my mouth.

I couldn't eat them fast enough. The first sugary lick at the peak of the vanilla cone soothed the burn.

Sure, some kids at school called me "Porkchop," but I was too young to associate the cruel nickname with what or how much I ate. Food and weight were not yet related to each other. Nutrition facts seemed like a foreign language, and carbohydrates, proteins, and fats sounded like fancy scientific terms. I ate what I wanted to eat, and just happened to be bigger than the other kids. I even faced the embarrassment of having my training wheels buckle under my large frame. However, the shame vanished under the golden arches.

As an early 90s kid, Velcro and elastic ruled my wardrobe. God bless neon track pants, right? Fashion trends changed alongside us. I wanted to wear jeans like all the other boys in my grade. However, I was too big for jeans in the regular section. My mom redirected my attention to a part of the store with piles of oversized garments and no mannequins: the husky section.

Husky is a word that still rattles me. The dictionary defines "husky" as strong and hefty. Well, one out of two ain't bad.

For the first time in my life, I felt the ostracization associated with body image. My large frame made me different, and not in a good way. "Different" for me meant the constant chafing of the denim against my thighs while my classmates appeared comfortable and relaxed in their jeans.

My classmates' bodies did not define them as mine did. On the first day of school, they greeted new friends with a clean slate. There was no baggage for them to hide. I, on the other hand, felt pre-defined. One look at my huskiness, and I was deemed "the fat kid."

But just as my dad knew how to bring happiness with a trip to McDonald's, he also knew how to talk through my problems with bullies. We covered various topics each evening in my parents' bed, ranging from funny jokes to who I wanted to be when I grew up (a horse jockey at the time). But we also discussed the more challenging moments in life while the rest of the world faded into the shadows. My dad's deep southern voice soothed like aloe after a burn.

From the outside it seemed like I had everything going for me. It was easy for me to make friends, and I spent every afternoon with neighborhood kids playing Power Rangers, shooting hoops, or setting up a lemonade stand. I also got all A's in class. Teachers fawned over my discipline and determination to do my best. The results from my state-required writing tests revealed I was writing at a high school level in third grade. My dad proudly told everyone he knew about his smart and talented son. A few years later I received an invitation to join the advanced math program. I had made a name for myself at Lake in the Hills Elementary School. Yet, the harsh words from a group of bullies tarnished the gold around me. The talks I had with my dad often revolved around what these kids would say about my weight.

"You're special, Jason," he said. "It doesn't matter what they think. One day you'll be big and strong. Only listen to the opinions of your friends, Nadine and Kelly, and ignore the rest."

I'd breathe deeply, feeling calmer. A smile emerged on my face as my dad placed his strong forearm between the pillow and my head. "You know what, Jase? I used to be a bit on the heavier side growing up, too," he said. "It's a phase. Once you hit your teenage years, you'll be driving around town with a slim figure and all the ladies hanging off you."

I couldn't wait. There was hope. My hero, who seemed perfect minus the occasional back pain from hard labor, was once like me and now everyone loved him. His encouragement deafened the insults of "Porkchop" and "Fatty," even if just for the moment.

Moments like these reminded me of why Dad was my hero. The oldest of eight, he spent his childhood moving between farms in rural Kentucky. His tan, tough skin revealed years of plowing fields and chopping wood. His smooth southern voice and tall stature commanded respect, like a modern-day Abraham Lincoln. Meanwhile, his bear hugs revealed the softie inside. Childlike energy beamed from his eyes every time he had a new joke or wild idea, like the time the Wood family gathered for a family reunion in the fall of 1996.

A rusty, run-down clubhouse in the middle of nowhere Kentucky came alive with laughter every time my father's cowboy boots walked through the door. "Gordon's here!" the family exclaimed as my aunts, uncles, and cousins flocked to see what my dad had up his sleeve.

The second day of the event always featured a white elephant auction. "Bid on that one, Daddy," I said, pointing to a yellow bag drowning in ribbons and bows.

"You got it, Jase." My dad could never tell me no.

"Twenty-five bucks, sold to Gordon," my aunt announced. The clubhouse grew silent, and my family awaited the reveal of the treasure inside that yellow bag.

"Well, looky here. I've got me a new set of bloomers and a brassiere. Darlene's going to be one lucky lady." Dad's tanned face wrinkled with glee. Laughter bounced off the cement walls as Dad held up a pair of ruffled women's underwear: off-white with plenty of lace. But Dad couldn't stop there. He never did. While the white elephant resumed, my father retreated to the bathroom.

Minutes later, from the back of the room I heard, "Howdy y'all! I think I might just keep these for myself." I turned around to see Dad walking the catwalk carved out by the long folding tables and relatives. The old man had put the bra and panties on over his western shirt and wranglers. The only thing louder than the laughter was the click of cameras capturing another silly moment presented by Gordon Wood.

Not only did Dad know how to have fun, but thanks to his experience on the farm, he also knew how to work. With only a middle school education, my dad left Kentucky in hopes of a better future and started an asphalt paving business from nothing.

Dad succeeded at everything he put his mind to, yet I was his proudest accomplishment. He waited forty-seven years for a son of his own. The man carried me up the stairs every night and all around town. Mom always said it's a wonder I ever learned to walk. My poor mother ended up sleeping in my bedroom since I stole her spot in the master bedroom, where my dad and I shared our nighttime talks.

Until, that is, our nighttime talks came to an end.

Our family first noticed something was wrong when Dad barely slept on our train ride to California. He winced in pain with each bump and twist of the railroad. It was his back again—the back pain his doctor assumed was due to my dad's line of work.

My dad used to chase me around the house playing "Tickle Monster." A week after the train to California, I found myself completing lap after lap between the kitchen and living room without a single tickle. I wasn't too concerned until the night my dad couldn't even make it up the stairs to bed for our bedtime chat.

When I was eleven, my robust, indestructible, super-hero dad met his kryptonite. We found out that the severe back pains he was experiencing were not the result of years of hard labor, but colon cancer. And by the time the doctors identified the cancer, it was too late.

Mom and I visited Dad daily in the hospital. The sterile whiteness of a hospital felt far away from the playgrounds of my childhood. In true Dad fashion, Dad masked his pain with a beaming smile when I was around. But the pale tint to his once bronze skin revealed something was wrong.

I blocked a lot of those memories from my mind. Yet, the beeps of the morphine drip and heart monitor still echo in my head. Those noises faded into the background one evening as Mom and I were leaving his room.

"Come on, Jase, we've got to get home now," she said, placing her hand on my shoulder. "Dad needs to rest, and you've got school and rehearsal tomorrow. Your fifth-grade play is coming up next week."

"Daddy, will you be able to make it to my play?" I asked from the side of his hospital bed. "I'm going to be Paul Revere!"

Mom and Dad exchanged looks, both knowing the truth would be too hard for me to hear. "I'll certainly try," Dad replied. "If not, Mom can record it for me!"

As we turned to exit the room, Dad grabbed my hand and whispered, "Jason, you're the man of the house tonight. Take care of your mom for me."

"You got it, Dad." I walked past the nurses' station with my chest puffed and chin up. My tiny world knew just one thing about the man of the house: he was brave and strong.

On a cloudy afternoon weeks later, I hugged my dad for the last time and watched him draw his last breath. My dad was a frail shell of himself; his lifeless and yellowed body terrified me. But I knew I had a promise to keep. Prior to the undertaker closing the casket days later, I whispered, "Daddy, I'll take care of Mom. Don't you worry. I've got this." Childhood was over. I was now the man of the house.

I tried to prove my manhood at school despite the constant jabs about my appearance. I held back tears and stared straight ahead, hoping I'd impress others with my resiliency. Like my father urged me, I wasn't going to let them get the best of me. But deep down, I knew that they were.

CHAPTER 2

ADOLESCENT AGONY

"**O**h damn, look at Fatty's boobs. Everything just jiggles. So gross, man."

I heard statements like this daily in that blue, humid middle school locker room. The smell of sweat and dirty socks matched the level of humanity around me. Amid a sea of average and muscular bodies stood my husky blob. My hands rattled every time I turned the dial on my locker because I knew the humiliation was about to commence.

"Fat ass!"

"Chubby!"

"Loser!"

I changed in and out of the gym uniform as fast as possible.

To avoid the locker room shame fest, I used my asthma as an excuse to sit out of gym class, or I'd go to the nurse before class so I could take my inhaler. An empty locker room felt much safer than one full of perfect bodies and big egos.

"Who cares what they think. You're smart and handsome to me," my mom said when I came home, dejected. But her words lacked the same connection I felt with Dad. A woman in her fifties does not feel very relatable to a boy entering puberty.

Don't get me wrong, though. My mom was quite the lady. Despite a rough childhood with neglectful parents, giving birth to my oldest sister in high school, going through two heartbreaking divorces before meeting my dad, and the numerous nights my mom sacrificed her own dinner so that my siblings could eat. My mom found joy in life in the little things. She didn't want fancy jewelry or perfume; Avon suited her just fine. Forget French bakeries; her eclairs from the Jewel-Osco were a delicacy. She'd take me on trips to the Hostess Outlet for half-priced Ho-Ho's and was always looking for the next garage sale.

I'm positive this was how my mom survived tough times. I'm lucky to have inherited that love of the small, simple things from her. It would prove crucial to the struggles that lay ahead for me.

My mom and I developed a unique relationship in the aftermath of dad's death because we had to rely on each other. We shared the grief. Dinner and vacations were just the two of us now, like our three-day train trips to visit my brother Mark in California. Mom and I spent the time in our tiny four-by-six room, playing cards and eating apple pie as the plains of Kansas and deserts of New Mexico whizzed past. We'd gossip about family members and laugh at fellow passengers on the train.

Mom did a fantastic job as the glue that kept our family together with her over-the-top events like holidays, complete with mountains of presents and plenty of cookies. With my four half-siblings and many nieces and nephews, this was important.

I will always cherish our family trips to the Wisconsin Dells, where we piled into the log boat ride at Timber Falls Adventure Park, laughing hysterically the entire way. And at the bumper boats, my mom was dubbed Bumper Boat Queen. It didn't matter if you were her kid, grandkid, or a stranger. Once she set sights on you, prepare for a wave of water coming your way!

As close as Mom and I were, Dad's death left a void. The insults from those around me echoed in my mind even as I made honor roll and achieved a new high score in bowling. The accomplishments didn't matter when I felt that the judgments of my peers mattered more.

While middle school was made up of middle-class white families who attended church every Sunday and took part in travel baseball leagues, high school represented a new beginning. There, in the exploding suburb of Chicago, kids from other schools with different backgrounds and personalities opened my eyes to a world where it was okay to be different. Well, at least to an extent.

I bounced around from clique to clique in high school, soon becoming friends with the popular kids, the musical kids, and the alternative bunch who were too cool for school. I loved striking up a conversation with the kid nearest to me in choir, often getting in trouble for disrupting the group. The lunch table doubled as my comedy stage to debut my latest satirical writing piece or share a new joke. My dad's outgoing personality had rubbed off on me.

However, one obstacle stood in my way: physical education. Before freshman year, Mom took me to a local store to order my school's gym uniform. They didn't have my size in stock, because I guess it's rare to have a 2XL student. I had to wait a couple of days; another painful reminder of my abnormal body.

The night Mom picked up my uniform, I took the bag upstairs and hid in my bathroom to change. I stood in front of the mirror. All I could see was how the yellow cotton t-shirt and brown mesh shorts revealed my layers of fat. I could already hear the taunts of "Porkchop" and "Sausage" echoing in my mind.

Determined to make a healthy change, I changed back into my pajamas and grabbed a bag of carrots from the kitchen before joining my mom for the first season of *Survivor*. I watched in awe as a fit contestant flexed for the audience. Their muscles bulged without an ounce of fat to conceal their strength. I could barely make it through gym class, and they could survive on a desert island.

I crunched the carrots like a machine, believing they would help me lose weight and look tan. I wanted to look like everyone else at school, and wear Abercrombie & Fitch for the first day. Instead, my body required the big and tall collection from Kohls.

After bingeing the entire bag of carrots, I was off to bed.

Halfway up the steps, my stomach tightened up. My mind jumped on a tilt-a-whirl, and my chest felt clammy. I crawled up the remaining steps. When I finally reached the cold yellow tiles of the bathroom, I was shaking. I could not stop thinking about the upcoming insults hurling my way in high school gym class.

"Are you okay, Jase?" my mom called to me up the stairs.

"Yeah, I'm fine," I said. "Must be a stomach bug or just too many carrots. Just go to bed."

Mom suffered from debilitating panic attacks, and now it was my turn. Anxiety dominated my mom's mind and body. Upon checking into a hotel in Indiana for a concert years prior, anxiety knocked the breath right out of her. Her trembling fingers clung to the front desk as I rushed to get a wheelchair. Alarmed by shallow breaths, the hotel clerk called the paramedics, and we spent the evening in the emergency room instead of the concert hall. Now I was experiencing those same sensations. But the man of the house would never admit that.

~

As anticipated, embarrassment reigned in the locker room for that first day of high school. In gym class, my locker was situated in a little cove of the locker room. Three walls of floor to ceiling compartments corralled at least ten sweaty teenage boys. A fat freshman sure feels out of place next to the muscular physiques of a senior.

"We need to get Wood a training bra," I heard amongst their chatter. And even when I couldn't hear the specifics of their conversations, I knew that the whispers and occasional roar of laughter was due to my appearance. Meanwhile, I stared at the brown tiles on the floor while fumbling to clothe as quickly as possible.

Why can't I just be average and fade into obscurity?

The walk down the hill to the track for gym class felt like a walk to my own execution each morning. "Pick up the pace, Wood," my gym teacher barked every time I huffed and puffed past the starting line. Eventually, I settled on making my own walking club composed of other individuals who detested running. We walked on the inside strip of the track between lane one and the sidelines of the football field. I jokingly referred to this as the French Fry Lane. For the badminton portion of class, I found myself paired with Luke, an arrogant kid who was never wrong and could do no wrong.

"Come on, Wood, try not to embarrass us too much against the girls," he muttered during a makeshift pep-talk on our way into the musty, old field house.

"Yeah, don't worry," I replied. "I got this."

I soon ate my words as the shuttlecock whizzed past my racquet more times than I could count. It felt like I took a dumbbell to the stomach each time I heard it bounce off the rubbery floor. The ladies on the other side of the net giggled at my futile attempts to run around the court.

"What the hell. Can you do anything right?" Luke asked. "God, you're so fat and lazy, man. I'm asking for a new partner; this isn't even fun." Throwing down his racquet, Luke stormed off.

"Oh, come on. It's just a stupid game," I said, forcing a chuckle to mask the pain.

Man, if I could have just one more talk with dad.

Around this time, I started to doubt Dad's advice. I was not losing the weight and slimming down like he said he did in his teenage years. Was I doing something wrong? I wanted to excel in everything, including sports. Sure, I was one of the best in my bowling league, but no one saw that as a macho sport. My high school only had a women's bowling team, not a men's. I wanted to be a tough guy, so I gave up bowling. Meanwhile, my self-doubt grew in tandem with my waistline.

CHAPTER 3

TIME FOR CHANGE

One summer evening just before sophomore year, my mom, sister, baby niece and I seated ourselves for dinner at a local family restaurant. It was there that I had a front-row seat to the illuminated pie case near the host station. Within moments of seeing it, I envisioned the slice of flaky crust and sugary filling I would eat after my meal of chicken strips, tater tots, a bowl of chili, and cornbread. After dinner, I asked for a slice of pie for the road.

"Wow, Jase, you sure ate a lot of unhealthy food," my sister scoffed. "You need to be careful so that you don't run into health problems. Maybe you should consider cutting back."

This was the first time a family member said something about what I was eating. In the past, my weight was just the elephant in the room. Most family members brushed it off or didn't talk about it. This comment about food especially hurt coming from my sister.

Lori is fourteen years older, the cool older sister. Her laugh would explode from her perfectly painted face, which was framed by flowing brunette hair. She was a strikingly beautiful person with the personality to match.

Lori used to treat me to special outings at the Applebee's or TGI Friday's bar. I'd order my Shirley Temple and munch on some potato skins while laughing the night away with her. Whether it was a funny song on the radio or something our mom said, we always had something to laugh about.

We're fourteen years apart, which meant she was closer in age to my peers' parents than my own mother. My friends loved it when Lori was our chaperone on school field trips. The most memorable moment was at the Brookfield Zoo, where my friends and I noticed a pair of wolves mating. "Look at how horny they are," my sister whispered to our group, trying to stifle her infectious laughter. My group of guy friends laughed their butts off and continued to talk about the incident the rest of the bus ride home.

Now, however, my sister and I were approaching different points in our lives. She was happily married with a baby, and heavily involved in church and caring for her family. I, on the other hand, was strapped in tight to the roller coaster of high school: a kid one day, an adult the next with the loss of my dad.

And that night, after the restaurant, my mind zeroed in on my weight as I devoured my slice of custard pie in the confines of my Jacksonville Jaguars-themed bedroom. Every gelatin-like bite of egg, sugar, and spice tasted of embarrassment as I berated myself, triggered by my sister's words.

Look at you, you Fatass. Look at those football players on the wall. They're real men. This can't go on any longer. You must fix this.

Little did I know, a "fix" was about to come.

A few weeks later at lunch, my friend mentioned she was going to check out Weight Watchers. My sister-in-law had just done it herself and praised the program. I figured it wouldn't hurt to check it out.

"Mom, will you drive me to Weight Watchers tonight?" I asked later that evening.

"Sure, but are you positive this is something you want to do?" she asked. My mom and I ate out nearly every night because she preferred not to cook, and I didn't care for her cooking. The woman mixed ketchup with ground meat and called it tacos. I figured she was just worried that Weight Watchers might impact our nightly dinners. I reassured her that I just wanted to learn more.

An empty storefront in a nearby strip mall was converted into a Weight Waters meeting place once a week, ironically situated between a Domino's Pizza and a Dairy Queen. Talk about temptation. That Tuesday night, I joined the Weight Watchers members lined up outside while freshly baked pizza wafted from Domino's. I wanted pizza, but I knew it would soon be off-limits. It would be one sacrifice of many on my journey to a better body. The word "sacrifice" made a home within my mind and heart.

Why do I have to give up foods I love when my friends can eat whatever they want and still be skinny? Why do I have to make yet another sacrifice? Wasn't Dad enough?

I followed the line into what looked like a voting booth—a small space lined by beige curtains with a silver scale. I pulled back the curtain to find a lady to greet me, her eyebrows raised in surprise to see a man here at the meeting. I stepped on the scale as the numbers bounced back and forth. They finally settled on 265.

I was obese, but I already knew that. Embarrassed, yet ready for change, I prepared myself to knock it out of the park. After all the members had gone through the weigh-in, I sat on a folding chair near the back of the room. Together we listened to advice from the group leader, a tiny lady with curly dark hair.

"We're in this together. You can do this," she said, clapping her hands and jumping up and down like a cheer captain. Next, fellow members walked to the front of the room to share their success stories. Despite the dirt-stained windows, matted-down carpet, and old creaky folding chairs, the women brought the room to life with their enthusiasm and smiles. They cheered their neighbors' successes with thunderous applause and a lot of whistling, encouraging us to push through adversity. I pledged to myself that I would be one of those success stories. Come hell or high water, I was going to succeed at this and earn their applause.

That night, I flipped through the two books Weight Watchers provided. The first one was thicker than our local phone book, with countless restaurants listed. Every menu item had points assigned. I quickly learned what I could and could not eat at McDonald's. And my lifelong addiction to Coca-Cola had to end. Too many points! The second book was smaller and consisted of common groceries.

I carried these books with me everywhere I went so I would always be aware of how many points I was consuming. At that time, I was allowed twenty-eight points. But this super honor roll student did the best he could to stay well below that number. Fewer points meant faster weight loss.

My philosophy went against what our group leader encouraged. "You should always eat your allotted points," she said. "Remember, an occasional day over your point limit would be perfectly fine." But I wanted to overachieve, so I kept my approach secret. The first week culminated in a weight loss of thirteen pounds.

"Did anyone lose more than five pounds this week?" the leader asked.

"I did," I said, smiling. I announced my thirteen-pound accomplishment.

The thunderous round applause and "Woo-hoos!" bounced off the white walls. When the leader handed me a pin for that week's loss, I realized I could earn praise and erase my imperfections by controlling what I ate.

I thrived under the challenge of counting points. I studied the materials provided and assigned a number to every food. Foods were not necessarily "good" or "bad" at this point. They just had number values, and I needed to find the correct equation for the day.

Six pounds here, three pounds there . . . each week was another exhilarating release of fat and shame. I also started to skip lunch and force myself to use the bathroom before weighing in to decrease the number on the scale.

"Wow, look at you, Jason!" my friend Aimee exclaimed as I got out of the car for a Friday night outing with friends. "I'm so impressed. You are doing such a good job on your diet."

When I placed my order for a fruit plate with a bun-less hamburger patty order that night, I hesitated, but only because my typical go-to French Dip with fries sounded damn good.

"Whoa, dude, you have some incredible willpower," my friend Steve remarked. "Look at Wood getting in shape." Hearing these words from a basketball jock boosted my confidence and determination to succeed at this diet.

"It really shows. You've lost so much weight," our friend Melissa chimed in. "Way to go! We'll have to go clothes shopping."

The rest of the table indulged in grilled cheeses, fries, and slices of pie. My fresh fruit, plain beef patty and cottage cheese lacked the same savory smells of their dishes, but it tasted mighty fine after hearing their praise.

A few weeks later I visited my dad's family side of the family in Kentucky. My aunts showered me in hugs and kisses.

"I'm happy for you. You are so much healthier now," Aunt Loretta said. "Your daddy would be proud, hun."

The trip was a whirlwind of praise. I smiled on my way home as I reflected on the opportunity to show off my new body and new clothes.

Lower numbers meant a gold star for the day. I could have a good day and take pride in myself. A stagnant number motivated me to work harder, while a higher number equaled failure. Higher numbers were rare back then. My infatuation with watching my weight was born.

While supportive and happy with the healthier me, my mom offered words of caution. "Don't go too extreme or be too hard on yourself, Jason," she said. "You're still a growing boy."

"You're just upset that I don't eat Hostess cupcakes for breakfast every morning with you anymore," I replied. "Or that I won't indulge in a Quarter Pounder with cheese. I'm healthier now, Mom."

I reached my goal weight in six short months. Shopping trips with my friends Katie and Kristen morphed from the boring Husky section to Abercrombie and American Eagle. Finally, my wardrobe was no longer oversized Hanes shirts and sweatpants. I could wear what the cool kids wore.

My childhood shame and embarrassment transformed into pride and accomplishment. For years, this feat defined who I was. Everywhere I went, I touted my weight loss. I felt accomplished and valued, unaware a fuse had been lit.

CHAPTER 4

ADULTING SUCKS

Following high school graduation, I moved to the upper peninsula of Michigan to attend Northern Michigan University. I was eager to start my life as an adult. However, the thought of additional education didn't appeal to me. I partly used college as a cover to escape, so I decided not to attend classes that fall. I knew I had my dad's asphalt-paving company waiting for me when I turned twenty-five. I looked forward to the challenge and the opportunity to carry on my father's legacy.

My townhouse sat on the remains of an old Air Force Base on the outskirts of civilization, which contributed to my feeling of isolation. College was outside of my comfort zone without the friends I grew up with and in a place hundreds of miles away from home.

What if I can't make new friends? What if the other guys laugh at me?

Ironically, the decision not to attend classes made it difficult to make new friends. I passed my days by scrolling through a brand-new site called Facebook.

The home pages of friends' Facebook pages revealed pictures of them playing frisbee in tree-lined quads and playing beer pong at home game tailgates. It was a far cry from my typical Friday night of eating cold pizza and watching sports alone. My friends and I frequently chatted over instant messenger, but a void remained.

Mom and I talked over the phone every day. This was the first time in her sixty-three years that she lived by herself. I worried about her health and often felt guilty for leaving her alone.

"Do you have any fun birthday plans?" she asked. "I wish you were here so we could celebrate."

"Yeah, Mom, of course. I'm going out with some new friends, and I have a fun night planned," I lied. In reality, I had no plans. I could have spent the evening on the phone with my mom and would have loved every minute of it, but pride got the best of me.

A few weeks later, I returned to Illinois for a cousin's funeral. While driving back to my mom's house for dinner with my mom and aunt, another driver blew a stop sign and t-boned my Chevy Avalanche. The impact sent my knees on a collision course with the dashboard, while my head kissed the windshield.

I spent months confined to the couch, which meant my Michigan experiment was over. Mom welcomed me home with open arms. During my recovery from the accident, the self-critical thoughts crept back in. What would I do with my life now? Yes, I could inherit Dad's company upon my twenty-fifth birthday, but that seemed like an eternity away. What would I do until then?

I felt the familiar pang of loneliness each night as I sat on the couch, scrolling through social media only to see more pictures of my friends continually moving on with their lives. My attempt at independence led to loneliness, isolation, and stagnation. And now, this car accident set me back even further. I had lost weight to fit in, but here I was again, feeling like an outcast.

One afternoon my buddy Nate mentioned he was going to a hiring event for a new family-style chain restaurant in the suburbs of Chicago, a place known for its ice cream creations and cheddar cheese chowder soup. I had fond memories of Monday nights there as a kid when the clown made balloon animals, so why not apply?

A couple of interview questions later and I had my first job as a host and server alongside an interesting cast of characters. This felt like a sequel to high school, except this time, I would define myself. My weight no longer could. I got to be the cool popular guy at work.

I worked the day shift at Colonial, which gave me plenty of time to stare out the door at my old stomping grounds. I longed for the days when I could just call up my friends and get together for a night of ghost hunting or video games. My mind also drifted back to my failed experiment at independence in the upper peninsula of Michigan.

Missing my high school crew, I turned to my co-workers to fill the void. These people were much more into drugs and alcohol than my high school friends. I tried marijuana for the first time and started smoking cigarettes.

You're just doing what the cool kids do. It's what you're supposed to do at your age.

My new life didn't mix well with my old friends. When I went to visit my friend Kelly in college for an overnight at a motel room, I spent the entire night stoned.

"Are you really smoking in here?" Kelly asked, appalled. "They'll call the cops or kick us out."

"Kelly, I paid for the room," I replied, annoyed. "I'll do whatever I fucking want." They were just jealous that I was enjoying life now and not absorbed in the demands of college, I thought. Other people were engaged in this sort of rebellion, so why couldn't I?

But my friends weren't the only ones who noticed the change. My sister Lori started searching my room on a regular basis for drugs and paraphernalia.

"I just don't know who you've become, Jase," she said one night. "You were such a good kid."

The first time I got drunk was at my buddy Eric's house. One of my co-workers had some Vodka so we figured we'd make a couple screwdrivers. They went down smooth—too smooth. I ended up calling my mom around midnight.

"Mom . . . This is, is ah, Jason. I'm so sorry. I drank lots of Vodka. I don't feel good. I'm sorry. I'm sorry . . ."

"Well, thank you for telling me, Jase," she replied. I was surprised to hear that her tone was soft. "Don't drive anywhere. Just stay there and come home in the morning when you're sober."

Despite my mom's gentle response on the phone the night before, I arrived home that morning, fearing a harsh lecture. Instead, I entered the family room to find Mom in her cozy tan recliner with a smile on her face. "Drank too much last night, didn't you?" she said, trying to hide her knowing smile. "Hop in the car, and let's grab some lunch. Maybe some soup and crackers will help you feel better."

My mom seemed to know I was going through a rough time and coped by drinking and partying. She was going through struggles of her own. I got the sense she wanted me to enjoy life and not worry too much about her.

But there was a lot to worry about. Like my dad, she had bouts of cancer in her lungs during my high school years. It didn't amount to the same fate as my dad, but by the time I was out partying and drinking, she began to experience severe headaches, dizzy spells, and weakness. Our primary care physician said her condition was just an ear infection and stress—stress, my family declared, I was bringing on. After all, I was the one living with her.

"Jason, it's up to you to care for your mother," my cousin said one afternoon. "Your drinking and smoking is stressing her out."

As frustrated as I was with this accusation, I wondered if I really was the one to blame. The worst of our fears gave us an answer a few days later. I found my mom sitting in her recliner with her head in her hands a day after going in for her yearly lung cancer scan.

"Mom, what's wrong?" I asked, standing paralyzed at the kitchen counter. "Did the doctor call with the results?"

My mom turned her head, her eyes brimming with tears. Her entire body trembled, making her curly hair bounce with fear. Her look said it all.

"Fuck no. Not again. I can't do this. I can't!"

I ran out the back door off the kitchen. Once on the deck, I screamed while tears cascaded down my face. When was enough, enough?

My dad's words returned to me at that moment: "You're the man of the house now, Jase."

I had to hold in the emotion. I had to be strong for my mom, and for my family.

Later that afternoon, my mom, my siblings, and I discussed surgery with the doctor in a small, cramped consultation room. We were all grieving, but my sibling had a spouse and children at home. Mom was my home.

Cancer inflicts not just physical harm but also emotional and mental pain. Mom's brain cancer diagnosis divided us like the scorching sun on dried earth. This event magnified the fact we were at different phases in our lives. My oldest sister would soon be a grandma, my middle siblings were starting families of their own, and I was just a

19-year-old kid figuring out life. Loneliness and fear consumed me. My family disapproved of my decisions. Even a part of me disapproved, but I had nothing else to cling to—until I realized I could find solace in maintaining a strict diet. This, after all, was my prized accomplishment.

Mom's surgery took place in late August. She then spent several weeks in the hospital and rehab. Once she returned home, I assumed responsibility for her care. This meant assisting her to the bathroom, changing her urine-soaked sheets, and ensuring she had something to eat.

I watched cancer ravage my mom's body in the same room where it robbed me of my father eight years earlier. I didn't have time to think of the pain I was going through. I couldn't show that, anyway, though. I was the man of the house and needed to prove it. Mom came first. I made that vow to dad before his death. I was the man of the house.

This meant I was on call for Mom all day. One afternoon, when we lost electricity following a powerful thunderstorm, I rushed home from work to help connect mom's backup oxygen tank. I found her sitting in her recliner gasping for air.

"Oh hon, thank goodness you're here. I didn't have the strength to get the tank from the closet."

"It's alright, Mom. I brought you home some ice cream. Gotta keep you fed."

I helped connect the new hose and then assisted her to the downstairs bathroom. I canceled my plans and stayed with her because I didn't know if we'd have to get a motel room for the night.

"The tank will only last for six hours, Mom. I'm going to run to Crystal Lake and grab some dinner for us. If the electric doesn't come back on soon, we'll need to go somewhere for the night."

In my mind, I didn't know how I'd transport her but knew I'd find a way if I needed to. Luckily, the power was restored when I got back home. Events like this became a common occurrence as Mom's condition deteriorated.

One evening, my close friends Katie and Heather invited me to go out to a club for a brief respite. When I say club, I'm referring to one of those teeny-bop clubs where the bar sells diet coke and sparkling water while teens dress to the nines in their Hollister and Abercrombie & Fitch. And every guy, including myself, had frosted tips. We were not heading out for VIP bottle service.

My oldest sister Holly, a nursing school student, offered to spend some time with Mom that night to give me a chance to get out and scream-sing Britney at the top of my lungs surrounded by my best friends.

But halfway to the club, my cell phone rang.

"Mom is dying, and you're acting selfish and irresponsible," my sister Lori said, seething. "You should be spending all your time with her. She won't be around forever. Instead, you're partying with your bad friends."

The car grew silent as my friends took note of the situation.

"Lori, I'm only nineteen," I said, my heart pounding. "This has been a lot to handle. Where have you been?" In fairness, Lori was busy with her own young family, but I wanted a life, too.

"I'm so disappointed in you," Lori said, ignoring my words. "I don't know who you've become."

I held back tears as I hung up the phone, trying to play it cool in front of my friends. But my shield of honor cracked. I'd always been the good kid. I loved my family. I needed approval. I wanted to impress others and be liked. These words from my childhood idol and mentor destroyed me.

"Wow, Jason. I'm so sorry you have to deal with her," my friend Katie said. "You're doing the best you can. You deserve one fun night."

But their words couldn't fix the hurt. No amount of dancing or laughing with friends that evening could take away what I was feeling, now. It would be a feeling I'd continue to carry for nearly two decades.

Three weeks later, the Sunday after Thanksgiving, Mom joined Dad. My heart, which I didn't know could feel more broken than it already did, shattered with the final beep of the heart monitor.

Lori served as executor and lightning rod. We rarely saw eye to eye. We were both grieving the loss of our mother, just in different ways.

And I couldn't escape the words of Lori's phone call.

You're a disappointment, Jason.

You're selfish, Jason.

You'll regret this, Jason.

A lengthy and heated estate battle commenced following Mom's death. I saw my dad's blood, sweat and tears go in the pockets of lawyers. Even his business, which was originally supposed to become mine in a couple of years, was sold. I not only lost my parents, but I lost my chance to preserve and carry on my dad's legacy.

Day by day, I also lost pieces of my childhood home. I often awoke to the shuffling and banging downstairs of my siblings and their spouses removing furniture and art by the carload from the house.

I stayed curled up in bed in my room, a hole growing larger in my chest as "home" transformed into an empty house. And then, partly due to our falling-out and my sister Lori's mistrust, I was ushered out of the house several months before it was sold. I found an apartment about thirty minutes away with a view of a hospital and dumpsters.

For the first few weeks of the move, my friend Stephanie stayed with me. She was there while I threw picture frames and yelled about how unfair my situation was. Sometimes, I would send a cryptic text about ending it all and speed off in my car to get away. One night, I threw myself down the stairs in front of my friends. I wanted to confirm they cared about me. I didn't really want to die, but I wasn't all that excited about the prospects of living, either. I needed someone, anyone, to tell me they loved me or that I mattered.

One night I spoke with a crisis counselor who told me that my problems weren't all that bad. "Just look at those poor folks in New Orleans," he said. "Katrina was much worse than what you're going through." My heart sank and my eyes welled up with tears.

You're a disappointment, Jason.

You're a failure, Jason.

You destroyed your family and your life, Jason. Do you regret it all yet?

The future felt like an unattainable illusion. There was no time to think about a year from then or even the next month. Life became a simple game of survival. My dad's company was gone, college seemed unaffordable, and my family felt like the enemy. I focused on delivering pizzas and trying to keep up with rent.

How could Mr. Super Honor Roll turn out to be a deadbeat?

I'll probably just work in food service the rest of my life.

I started staying up until four or five in the morning by myself getting high and watching YouTube videos. They seemed to be the only thing that could make me laugh and forget about the estate battles, stolen legacies, and tarnished memories.

One day off from work, I sat on the couch surrounded by unpacked moving boxes and felt an intense contraction in my abdomen, followed by gurgling. The sun was setting, and I realized I hadn't eaten all day. Normally, on days that I worked I ate pizza since it was free. Rent and other bills prevented me from affording much else. I had lived in that apartment for almost eight months, and had only gone grocery shopping once. I lacked an appetite and a desire to learn how to cook. In the setting sunlight, I propped myself up on the couch and embraced the pain.

Wow, physical pain numbs the other pain but is much more manageable and comes with benefits. Finally, something I can control. Something I am good at.

CHAPTER 5

MR. TOUGH GUY

My best friend at the time, Kyle, was big into mixed martial arts and working out. He was a strong guy with no emotion. Arrogance radiated from his dark, brown eyes, while a selfish sense of pride guided each word from his lip. He inspired me to do the same. I wanted to be one of the guys, like him.

Raised by a widowed mom from age eleven, I never felt very masculine according to society's standards. Anytime a "tough guy" paid attention to me, I became fixated on being just like them and spending all of my time with them. I'd often get jealous when a new girlfriend came along and stole my bro-time. There were many bro-mances before Kyle, but his friendship left the most profound impact on early-twenty-something Jason.

Pushing my true friends aside, I pursued this new lifestyle and friendship. I was eager to latch onto anything or anyone that felt like direction or value. At the time, this meant lifting weights and embracing Kyle's arrogance. That, I believed, would make me feel valued and become the man society expected me to be.

Kyle worked at the local gym and would let me in before opening. I loved this setup because I could avoid being seen by the fit dudes and prevent a repeat of high school gym class. I usually rode the exercise bike for thirty minutes, followed by a half hour on the treadmill. The steeper the incline, the more accomplished I felt. This was followed by several mile walks throughout the day.

Kyle even helped me set up a workout room in the guest bedroom of my new place complete with weights and a bench. He was there to "encourage" me with comments like, "Man up, Wood," and "Come on, Pussy, is that all you got?"

Kyle eventually revealed his true colors. He was simply my friend because I paid for everything including mixed martial arts lessons at a local gym. My self-doubts and insecurities made me an easy target. As soon as the little inheritance I received ran out, so did he, but not after leaving me completely broken.

One lasting remnant of this toxic friendship was my newfound obsession with working out. I was no longer recording thirty-minute miles with constant side stitches and a high school gym teacher barking orders. Now, skinny Jason could run without feeling sick. But it seemed that no matter how hard I tried, I could not be the man society expected me to be, at least from the physical and macho perspective. I believed those two things went together like peanut butter and jelly. The more muscle you have, the more manly you are and vice versa. And even though I pushed my body to the limits in the gym, I failed to provide it with the nutrients for growth.

My diet consisted of a bowl of Special K Cereal in the morning, a peanut butter and jelly sandwich for lunch, and a bowl of oatmeal with a banana for dinner. I justified my regimen with excuses about how I couldn't afford anything else or didn't know how to cook. The food rules seemed to provide stability amid the turbulent times.

The increased exercise and lack of proper nutrients resulted in a drastic weight loss. My clothes became baggier, and my ribs grew more pronounced. The scale bottomed out to my lowest numbers thus far. Friends would say things like, "Oh my God, you're so skinny!" or "Oh, you should eat more." Gym rat, oatmeal-loving Jason. I would just tell myself that they were jealous that they couldn't be this skinny or have the willpower to do this.

The embers of an eating disorder were beginning to glow.

CHAPTER 6

RELOCATION, EVICTION, AND DARKNESS

I moved ten times across the Chicagoland suburbs in my early twenties. Sometimes I slept on friends' couches. Other times I lived in motel rooms.

The restlessness of my physical location matched that of my mind. My weight and diet followed suit. There were times I wouldn't eat for an entire day because I had little money and couldn't justify spending anything on food. It didn't help that the electricity had been shut off. I had no stove, microwave, or refrigerator for food prep and storage.

No electricity meant no hot water. Except for an occasional shower at my best friend's house, I usually just bathed myself with a washcloth. In the mornings I dressed in a dark bathroom before I headed to the city for work.

Half my paycheck went to the train ride downtown. I literally worked to pay for the ride to and from work. I debated finding a job closer to home, but not many employers were looking to hire someone without a college degree in the middle of a recession.

I often rerouted food funds to cigarettes and a tallboy beer from the gas station across the street because they numbed my hunger and the anxiousness, if only for a moment. Healthy food is not cheap, nor is eating out.

Cigarettes became my comfort food. They were my biggest personal expense, but they killed two birds with one stone. The temporary buzz calmed a world spinning out of control and suppressed my hunger. I hated myself for taking up the same habit that aided in my parents' deaths. And I knew gas station pizza and nicotine wasn't good for me, but the fear of returning to my childhood chubbiness haunted my mind.

I slept on the pull-out couch in my apartment since a real bed was out of my price range. The white walls of that 500 square-foot apartment closed in on me as the days passed, and the smell of nicotine and dog urine cast a shadow over my soul.

I spent hours by the sliding door, peering out at the parking lot and building across from me. My neighbors, hosting game night with friends on their deck, seemed to live in a whole different world from the one their neighbor across the street was living in.

I stayed home most nights, unable to afford to go out and too embarrassed to see my close friends. I worried about what they would think of me. I felt like I was a disappointment and didn't want to hear one more remark about how skinny I looked. My only outing was to the racetrack each Saturday afternoon; the same racetrack I went to with my dad. Now, I only had enough money for a beer and a couple $2 bets. Those summer afternoons at Arlington Park were my only escape from the daily grind of work, sleep, and worry. But the main reason I went to the racetrack was to feel close to my dad.

I often sat on the benches overlooking the track and stared off at the weeping willow trees that lined the backstretch. Dad's voice seemed to whisper to me through the trees, telling me to just hang on.

By this point, all ties with my siblings had been cut. The estate was just about settled. The only contact I had with family was a weekly call with my Aunt Loretta back in Kentucky.

"Aunt Loretta, I can't even pay my bills," I said over the phone one night. "I've been left with nothing. All I do is work but I just can't get ahead."

"Oh hon, I hate this for you," she replied in her gentle southern voice. "Your daddy would not have wanted this. Just remember God never gives us more than we can handle. I'll talk to Uncle Russ and send you some money if we can."

"I promise I'll pay you back one day," I said. "I just don't know when or how."

"Don't worry, sweetie. We just have to keep that roof over your head. Plus, I'm worried about you. You were so skinny last time you came to visit. Please make sure to eat."

"Yes, I'm eating. Can't afford much, but I try to eat when I feel like it. Love you."

Medical bills racked up during this time from frequent doctor visits. When you watch your parents die from diseases that reveal themselves as back pain or an earache, you become paranoid that the slightest ache and pain is death knocking at the door. Indigestion, a headache, or a tingle in my toe often led to a trip to the emergency room.

About six months after moving into my apartment in Lisle, I walked off the train one night from work and was greeted by the yellow eviction notice on my apartment door. I swallowed my pride and moved in with my friend's grandparents for two months. I'm forever grateful for their kind gesture. The move took me away from my friends but allowed me to get back on my feet.

I found solace and control in the growing set of rules around food. Weight loss was the only thing I was proud of, and that meant I was nothing more than the digital numbers on the scale. My daily menu consisted of a footlong Sweet Onion Teriyaki Sandwich every day from Subway. I ate one half for lunch and one half for dinner. Five bucks was all I could afford, and the 300 calories in each half were all I would allow myself: no chips, no fancy toppings, just the meat, and bread. If I felt frisky, I would sneak in a banana or slice of melon for dessert; however, the goal was to go to bed hungry. Hunger pains numbed the other pain.

The weekends, however, brought endless amounts of fast food and alcohol. I upgraded from the dollar menu to the extra value menu for a Saturday night delight. This became my reward for starving all week.

CHAPTER 7

THE UNKNOWN TRUTH

"**W**ait, what? No way you were obese."

These were the common reactions I got when I told others of my childhood with Weight Watchers.

"Yeah," I would reply. "And to keep the weight off, I only eat three meals a day. No snacking. No dessert during the week. And absolutely no eating before bed."

The thought of an eating disorder never crossed my mind. I still ate food when I could afford it and I never threw up. I hate throwing up. According to school and media, those seemed like the only two behaviors to determine an eating disorder. Plus, guys don't have eating disorders.

I praised willpower when those hunger pains hit every morning around ten and afternoon around three. I figured most people faced a high amount of anxiety around food, so I wasn't alone. It was just something people didn't talk about.

Doctors didn't pick up on unhealthy habits either. "Your BMI is perfect," my primary care physician would tell me. "You're one healthy, good-looking guy Mr. Wood. You must have all the ladies!"

The nurses never hesitated to comment, either: "Are you a runner? Your vitals are incredible."

"Sure am," I lied while laughing to myself. My ego gladly accepted the perceived compliment.

See, Jason, your quirky diet and food rules are making you the epitome of perfect health. Keep it up!

Around this time, I came to terms with a groundbreaking revelation about myself. I thought about how my closest friends tended to be females. My struggle with masculinity was a significant force behind my self-criticism and lack of confidence. I blamed the void of a male authority figure in my life. I blamed my skinny frame and lack of muscles. I blamed the voices that haunted me from childhood about being fat and husky.

I was fascinated with men and whenever a "cool guy" showed any semblance of friendship or interest in me, I clung to him like a bad toupee. I needed that male companionship and approval. At the time, I didn't see that it could be something more than that.

Curiosity took advantage of me one Memorial Day when I started talking with a guy on Craigslist. After realizing we both wanted to drink and eat a McChicken sandwich, we decided to meet up. My fingers trembled as I typed in the address of my apartment. My roommate was at her boyfriend's place for the night, so I had the place to myself.

I spent the next twenty minutes pacing the dirty carpeted floors.

What will he think of me? What will we do? Oh my God, what if he is a murderer?

When I heard a knock on the door, I looked through the peephole to see a skinny figure who matched the picture he sent. *Okay, a good sign.* My heart raced as I laid eyes on a skinny blond guy standing on my front porch.

After we nervously exchanged greetings, the two of us walked up the stairs to the balcony of my room which overlooked the apartment complex's parking lot. Sipping on our brews, we talked about our favorite artists (Britney, Gaga, and High School Musical!). And when I found out that he worked at Boston Market, I was sold on the guy. Free mac and cheese, baby!

Mr. Craigslist was a nice guy; someone I wanted to know more about. And this was much more than a friendship connection. My fascination with males and my longing to be like them evolved into an attraction.

That evening, nervous energy erupted like a firework as Mr. Craigslist leaned over and kissed me. My unrestrained glee within formed goosebumps from head to toe. I tend to jump to conclusions quickly, but at that moment, I knew I was gay.

There was nothing to hide, even though I never really considered myself living in the closet. If so, I was in the closet from myself as well! I associated my interest in the male body with my desire to look like them, blind to the fact it could be a genuine attraction. Plus, I've always been a huge sports fan. The club scene and other stereotypical gay activities matched my definition of hell. I didn't fit the stereotypes, but as I would later learn, this also applied to other aspects of my life.

I saw a future of happiness and love again. And to think about the future at all was a welcome sight. I shared the good news with my friends right away.

"Kelly, there's something I want to tell you. I realized a couple of days ago that I'm gay."

"Oh hell, we already knew that. But good for you!"

"Kate, I'm gay. I'm dating a guy."

"Oh my god! Yay! That's so exciting, and now we get free Boston Market!"

I climbed a hill to come out of the closet to my friends, but the Rocky Mountains lay ahead with my family. The Wood family are God-fearing Southern Baptists. They lived hundreds of miles away, so I could just avoid them for the most part.

I stopped traveling to Kentucky; it was self-imposed isolation for my own good. I cut back on the number of phone calls I made and often used work or lack of funds as my excuse for not seeing them more often. When asked about my relationship status, I'd respond with one of my female friend's names and make up some story. But the pain and loneliness from not being able to be my authentic self stung deep.

I became an expert in hiding myself. First, the extra fat on my body through diet and exercise. Now, my sexuality. I made sure to keep my voice low and personality reserved around new people, professional settings, and family. I allowed myself to "let go" on nights out with friends. With the back and forth between hiding and revealing myself, I wasn't sure who Jason really was. And if the real Jason was weak or not good enough, I'd have to continue to hide him.

CHAPTER 8

FAMILY FALLOUT

A few months passed before I connected with a cousin on my mom's side of the family via Facebook. Jenny had always been an outsider in the family, a title I now seemed to share with her. She acknowledged how messed up the estate battle was and that she didn't believe the things my sister Lori had said about me being irresponsible and out of control. My face lit up when she invited me to join her family and my Aunt Nancy for Easter dinner. I viewed this as a potential turning point. Maybe the loneliness was over.

My cousin's dining room illuminated in the spring sun as we spent hours reminiscing about our family's Fourth of July shenanigans.

"Remember how your mom always arrived at one o'clock and sat between first and second base on the baseball field waiting on the fireworks?" Jenny laughed.

"And your daddy just thought the world of you, Jason," Aunt Nancy said, smiling. "He'd take you over to that carnival and spend a small fortune to win you a gigantic stuffed horse."

I laughed and smiled with them, all while happily shoveling in the delicious ham and potatoes. For dessert we had an oddly shaped bunny cake, my first semblance of a family in quite some time. My mom's side of the family loved those kitschy holiday food items. I sat there staring at that chocolate cake and laughed about how much joy it would have brought Mom.

After dinner and dessert, Aunt Nancy and I snuck out back for a cigarette and some one-on-one time. "J. Dubya," Aunt Nancy said, sitting down on the white bench overlooking the garden. I smiled at her use of my nickname again. "I think about your mom every day and how sad she would be to see you going through so much." The warm spring breeze tickled the delicate graying waves framing her face.

I nodded, looking down at my lap. "I've made mistakes, Aunt Nancy," I said. "I know I'm not perfect, but I'm not a bad person. I'm just tired of always fighting to survive. I miss my family."

"I know, hon. You're going through a lot right now. You're grieving your mom in different ways. But your Uncle Mike and I are very proud of the young man you've become."

I hugged Aunt Nancy's frail body, taking in the familiar smell of cigarettes and rose perfume. Tears threatened to burst forth the moment we hugged. She smelled like Mom.

My cousin Jenny and I kept in touch all summer. When fall came, I needed a place to stay because my roommate was moving in with her boyfriend at the end of our lease. I tried to find another roommate, but to no avail. My cousin offered to let me stay with her while I found something permanent, but on one condition: my beloved dogs, Daisy and Bullwinkle, could not come. These little white and brown chihuahua mixes were my family. We survived darkness and eviction together. But I needed to make this sacrifice to survive. I was thankful that my friend's grandparents offered to watch them.

I cried most of the car ride down to their temporary home. I cherished each pant and nose print on the passenger-side window. Daisy and Bullwinkle stayed in a room off the garage where my friend's grandfather kept his show dogs when they were in heat. There were plenty of fuzzy blankets and a dog bed to comfort them from the cement floor. I peered at Daisy and Bullwinkle through the chain-link kennel, vowing to be back soon.

~

I'd only been at my cousin's house for three weeks, most of that time spent in bed recovering from mono. Work wouldn't allow me to return until I saw my doctor the following week, so I went to my friend's house to work remotely—anything I could do to get away from my cousin's husband, Tony.

Tony lived up to that macho, tough-guy persona portrayed by Hollywood. His salt and pepper hair clashed with the redness of his leathery face. If you didn't know him, you'd think he was a used car salesman. At first, Tony greeted me with open arms. Then, the facade came off.

I invited my new boyfriend Marcus over one night. He was a cop and an all-around good guy. We had just started dating when I came down with mono, so it was great to be able to see him again. He suggested we watch a movie and relax on the couch since I was still recovering from my illness.

Shortly after Marcus arrived, we settled in on the living room couch. My cousin Jenny and her son were both at work that evening while I figured Tony was in another room of the house, working.

Marcus and I were half an hour into the movie when I heard thundering of footsteps into the garage.

"You," Tony said, ripping open the door and pointing at me. "Get outside. Now. We need to talk."

My stomach twisted into knots. Shaking, I followed Tony out back.

Once in the backyard, Tony pulled me to the side of the house. The rage on his face incited a fear that this could get physical.

"What the fuck do you think you're doing? Just taking advantage of all of us? Your sister is right about you, you shithead. What if your cousin wanted to watch TV tonight when she got home? How selfish and irresponsible. Grow up or get the fuck out."

In his eyes, it was tough love, but for me, I just needed love.

"I . . . I am so sorry," I said. I was stunned. I tried to wrap my head around what I did wrong, and how I could fix this. I had invited my boyfriend over. Maybe I should have asked, I thought. I should have known my place. I was just a guest.

"Tell Marcus to go home," Tony said.

"Yes, sir," I replied, my voice shaking.

But I couldn't escape trouble even when I met up with friends outside of the home. Out at the bar one Friday night, recovering from the previous Wednesday's ordeal, I felt my phone buzz. My cousin was calling, but I didn't answer. The noisy bar was no place for a phone call. The round of text messages I got moments later made me think otherwise.

"You're a thief. I'm going to kick your ass, you faggot."

"We're calling the cops."

"Get the fuck out of here. I'm pissing on your clothes."

Flabbergasted, I got up from the bar and pushed open the heavy wooden doors to call my cousin from the parking lot.

"What's going on?" I asked. "What happened?"

"You know exactly what you did, Jason. How could you do that after all, we've done for you?"

"No, what are you talking about? What's going on?" I asked, desperate.

"You stole $60 from your cousin, Johnny. Now return the money and get out," Jenny yelled.

I tried to tell them over and over that I hadn't taken any money. As a people-pleaser, even the thought of doing so made my stomach drop. But nothing would convince them. I finished the call by promising to be back in the morning to get my things.

Standing in the parking lot, I felt as if I had gotten the wind knocked out of me by a blindside tackle. How could my family think I would steal? I returned to the bar with my friends to explain the situation and asked for a place to stay that night. After a night of tossing and turning on my friend Kate's couch, I decided to call the local police for an escort to my cousin's house. The officer arrived and maintained the peace while my best friend and I quickly loaded up my clothes and miscellaneous items.

"I pissed on your clothes," my cousin's son told me as I walked past him to the car.

"How could you do this?" Tony spit. "Your sister was right about you. How could you hurt your family like this?"

Head down, under the safety of my friend and police officer, I threw my belongings in the car and got the hell out of there.

That event marked the end of a turbulent experiment trying to reunite with my long-lost family. I made the commitment to myself to never trust anyone again, including blood.

A year later, my cousin's son confessed via Facebook Messenger that he lied about the accusations that I stole his money. Apparently, he was jealous of me for having a boyfriend, while he was struggling with his own sexuality. Unfortunately, it was too late. The damage was done.

I moved in with my friend's grandparents in their rural farmhouse next. There, I just wanted to binge on comfort foods. Dad's McDonald's hypothesis sounded pretty good right now; perhaps an Extra Value Meal would do the trick. These urges fanned the flames of hatred and disappointment inside. I knew my one true strength was willpower around food, so I despised the fact I had these cravings.

My co-workers loved to order in for lunch every day and always invited me to join them. They'd snack on pizzas, hamburgers, and fries while I stuck to my low-fat, low-sodium one slice of turkey sandwich on whole wheat bread as a "special" treat. I allowed myself up to ten potato chips, the kettle-cooked kind of course, if the scale said I could.

Around this time, I also changed from oatmeal every morning to a granola bar and Diet Coke. If I filled myself up on the zero-calorie bubbly soda, then it could quell my hunger until lunch. The more diet soda I drank, the fuller I felt. It became the newest tool to my arsenal of staying thin and valuable.

While bouncing around from place to place, one constant remained: the scale. It dictated my feeling of self-worth as well as what I was going to eat that day. I knew it wouldn't leave me even if I wasn't always happy with what it said.

I began to see my weight creep up after weekend binges of pizza, beer, and doughnuts. While we may shove the same greasy delights down our throats on the weekend, friends seemed to do so with confidence and no guilt. I watched with envy as my friends and colleagues enjoyed pasta, burgers, and cookies. The fear of being "Porkchop" or "Fatty" again paralyzed me, so I stuck with my healthy foods like yogurt for breakfast and the occasional peanut butter sandwich for lunch. Even jelly, full of sugar, was too much for me now. I needed to lose as much as I could Monday through Thursday so I could try to enjoy those 3 a.m. burritos with friends on weekends without too much guilt.

CHAPTER 9

NEW BEGINNINGS VS. PAST MISTAKES

A little over a year after coming out and after my relationship with Marcus ended, a new guy in the mailroom at work caught my eye—a tall, dark temp with a deep, confident voice and an infectious childlike smile.

"Mari, I'm in love. I have to get him to notice me," I told my trainee-turned-close friend.

"Oh, my love, you two would be so cute together. He's a hottie." her eyes beamed behind her dark-rimmed glasses. "We're going to make this happen."

According to my Facebook stalking skills, Matt had lived all over the world, from Tokyo to Barcelona. He strutted around the office with a clear confidence in who he was. I learned through our casual cigarette breaks that he wanted to go into architecture and travel the world. I don't know if it was love at first sight, but I knew I wanted him in my life.

There was one big problem: I felt ashamed of my disaster of a life. Even though I was sleeping on a couch in my friend's grandparents' basement at the time, I kept the details from my co-workers. I just told them I was going through a transition, and this was temporary. After several months of saving up, I moved into the Red Roof Inn across the street from my new job. My own place. Two double beds, cable TV, and fresh towels. Yeah, I sure seemed like a catch, huh?

I dressed up for work every day, going a little bit further than the required business-casual look. Ties became my favorite fashion accessory, even though they weren't required. But shyness prevented me from saying much to Matt in person, so I resorted to Facebook messenger to ask him out.

"Hi, this is Jason from work," I wrote. "Would you like to grab lunch sometime?"

"Sure!" Matt replied. "You know you can swing by my office. I don't bite."

I wanted to kiss those beautiful words on the fuzzy computer screen.

Our first date took place in the bustling cafeteria of Chase Tower. Surrounded by suits and ties, Matt told me about his worldly travels. Meanwhile, I only shared what I wanted him to hear.

"I'm staying in the boondocks with my friend's grandparents but that's only temporary," I said. "I'm just in between places right now."

By this point, I had dated several guys, but Matt's maturity set him apart. I'll never forget the power I felt when he hugged me for the first time. He felt solid; not just muscular, but solid from the inside out. Our relationship grew, as did my hope for the future.

I slowly opened up to Matt about some of the problems in my life, like the estate battle, my fragile living situation, and the mounting debt I faced from medical bills. I feared losing him, and almost did just shy of our first anniversary.

A few years prior, on Christmas Day, I had been involved in a fender bender. No money meant no car insurance. The judge ruled I pay for damages and maintain SR-22 insurance for two years. I failed to make a payment, and my insurance lapsed. A few days later, I received a letter from the Secretary of State informing me that my license was suspended. Along with the suspension came a hefty fine. Living paycheck to paycheck doesn't leave much room for a four-figure fine. I evaded the law for a couple of years because I still needed to drive myself to work.

Then my luck ran out.

My office was literally across the street from the Red Roof Inn where I lived. However, it was a hot summer afternoon in Chicagoland—the kind where the humidity bathes you with just one step outside. I decided to drive to work that day to avoid the heat. Plus, I needed to stop at a nearby gas station after work for cigarettes and my large diet soda. I turned on the side road, which ran parallel to the motel, and saw a cop following me around the corner. My heart skipped a couple of beats. I proceeded past the motel en route to the gas station a few blocks away. Pulling up to a four-way stop, I stopped an extra five seconds longer. I devised a plan to pull into Wendy's parking lot, hoping the cop would go straight. Then I knew I'd be in the clear.

When I flashed my right turn signal, the cop car did as well. My sweaty palms clinched the steering wheel. While my eyes stayed fixed on the developments in the rear-view mirror, the red and blue lights screamed to life.

I frantically texted Matt. "Getting arrested. I'll be at the Naperville jail," I wrote.

My chest and stomach tightened as the officer approached my vehicle. He asked me to step out of the car and started applying the handcuffs. All I could think about were the rush hour commuters seeing this criminal get cuffed, with no understanding of the hell that led me there.

~

How could you be so stupid? Lori was right. You are a big, fat disappointment.

My wrists, sore from the cuffs, ached each time I dried a tear from my eye.

Several hours after sitting in a pink jail cell, Matt bailed me out. I could barely make eye contact with him when he asked, "What do we do now?"

"Well, we need to get a lawyer, I think. I have a court date in several weeks. And we have to get the car out of impound." That's when I began to panic. "Oh God, I can't afford all of this."

"It's okay," Matt said. "I'll help you pay for this as long as you pay me back at some point." It was a lot to ask from someone who was a stranger less than a year before.

A few days later we met with a lawyer, who eventually settled with the courts. Still, I lost my license for nearly a year.

"Can you drive me or pick me up?" became a common question for me to ask my friends. It never got easier to ask. I felt trapped inside my smoky prison cell at the Red Roof Inn.

Several weeks after my first court appearance, I received an ominous text from Matt: "Want to grab dinner tonight? We need to talk."

It was difficult to focus on work the remainder of the day. We decided to grab Chipotle for dinner that night. I wasn't very hungry since my stomach was in knots awaiting this dreaded conversation. Matt remained quiet throughout dinner, nibbling away at his overflowing burrito bowl. Small talk about work seemed to be the only topic of interest. By the time we left the restaurant, I wanted to throw up.

Why won't he say what he wants to say? This must be bad.

It wasn't until we returned to my hotel room when Matt finally shared his feelings.

"You know we're just moving in different directions right now," he began. "This has been so stressful on me. So, I think we need to take a break. I'll still help you with groceries and stuff, but I just can't handle everything else right now."

I sat there in shock.

Look at what you've done now. Your life is such a mess. Nobody will ever want to be with you. A total embarrassment and disappointment.

"I understand," I said. "I want nothing but the best for you." It felt like the right thing to say, but my heart shattered. I couldn't blame Matt. His life was going places. I felt like he deserved so much better than me.

True to his promise, Matt brought groceries to my door every Sunday. The first couple of weeks I asked him to just leave them at my door. I couldn't face looking at his beautiful dark eyes, the hazel eyes that once lit up my world.

The ice bucket in my room served as a refrigerator. Most of the time, however, I just tossed the food out. I wanted to waste away at that point—the skinnier, the happier. I lay in that cold motel room, with the light-blocking curtains closed. Here I was again, alone because of my own stupid mistakes.

Even though we might have broken up, Matt continued to visit me and take me on errands. That Thanksgiving, he drove an hour to pick me up from my friend's house. We took vacations together, including a much-needed break to Grand Rapids, Michigan. I confided in him when I had a bad day at work or just needed someone to cheer me up. Friends often asked if and when we were going to get back together. They saw that love is love. Finally, one night, Matt recognized it, too.

We were lying in Matt's bed looking out the window at the sparkling lights of the Chicago skyline, when he whispered, "I love you."

"What . . . what did you say?" I asked, stunned. I looked into his eyes, not truly believing this was the moment. "Did you really say that?"

Matt nodded, smiling. It was a feeling I hadn't had since my parents drew their final breaths so many years ago. Someone else could come into my life like this, and love me, too.

I was loved.

"I love you, too," I whispered. "I love you."

Our relationship grew stronger through these challenges. Matt was the Ricky to my Lucy, the Marge to my Homer. He was the anchor of our relationship that kept us grounded while always cooking up my next crazy antic. Matt helped stitch up the lingering wounds of years gone by. Life felt a lot more manageable with him by my side.

This was a blessing and a curse because it just gave my inner critics more to talk about.

CHAPTER 10

HOUSTON, WE HAVE A PROBLEM

Determined to be healthier and save some money, I put out my last cigarette on January 6, 2014. Breaking free of that dirty habit felt great, but it came with a cost.

Websites suggested self-love during the nicotine withdrawal process. For me, self-love meant bingeing on Chinese food and cupcakes. I no longer had the cigarette in my diet control arsenal.

My weight crept up a few pounds. The tighter fitting clothes felt suffocating as I got ready for work each Monday morning.

∼

Later that year, Matt accepted a job offer in Houston and asked me to move with him. We had never lived together. In fact, for the first time in my adult life, I had a steady income and stable living situation. Moving across the country, leaving my job, and living with someone posed daunting challenges. But I mostly worried about how I would maintain my strict intake regimen during the week.

Matt moved first to start work and settle in. I arrived in early December and soon realized this diet of mine would be trickier than feared.

My first grocery shopping excursion to HEB left me in tears. They didn't have the passion fruit Greek yogurt I ate every morning. In fact, I couldn't find it anywhere in town. And my go-to lunch of low sodium canned vegetable soup had different shaped noodles than I was accustomed to. Worst of all, Matt was upset that I didn't buy anything for him.

I felt so out of my comfort zone that I cried right there in the parking garage of our apartment complex. I even doubted whether I could make this new living arrangement work. All of this over a stupid yogurt variety.

Before the move, I ate frozen cheese ravioli for dinner every weeknight: no sauce, just some black pepper, and a spoonful of frozen vegetables. The scale approved, so I did as well. But I had to break my restrictive eating habits. I now had another mouth to feed at dinner. Plus, I didn't want Matt to make fun of me or think I was crazy for strict regimens. This left me distraught and out of sync for several weeks. I stayed unusually quiet and kept to myself. I'd drive around town to try and take my mind off my anxieties.

The kitchen and I were mortal enemies. I replaced my shield with an apron to feel like I could contribute to the house and our relationship. I started cooking dinner several nights a week.

I modified my habits to eat lighter during the day so I could have more calories and variety at night. The weekends were still mine. However, I couldn't escape Judge Judy whispering body insults and food critiques over my shoulder when I didn't follow my food rules.

Matt was the breadwinner, providing for us while I returned to school to finish my bachelor's degree. I wanted to go into sports communications because it combined my love of sports with my love of writing and talking. However, I quickly found myself feeling insufficient.

Jason, you're not a man. You are nothing. A disappointment.

I clothed these inner doubts with my arrogance and drunkenness, which not only affected me, but now Matt, too.

Right after arriving in Houston, we attended Matt's company holiday party. Architecture firms can put on a damn good event. The party took place at the River Oaks Country Club in Houston, where the streets lined with decorated mansions and perfectly landscaped yards.

I arrived in one of Matt's suits, too poor for my own. The night consisted of glass of wine after glass of wine. At one point, I asked the husband of the couple we were talking with to grab the bottle of wine when the bartender wasn't looking. He obliged, which probably contributed to my black out. The next thing I remember is waking up on the couch with part of the suit still on.

"You sure seem like you had a good time last night," Matt said, coming out of the bedroom.

"Oh no, what did I do?" I asked, head pounding.

"What didn't you do? I hope you didn't embarrass us too much." With that, Matt walked into the bathroom and closed the door. My heart hurt alongside my head with fear of what I'd done. This would not be the only time my drinking got out of control.

Around this time, a trip to the grocery store filled me with enough rage to complain for a week straight. I honked and cussed out fellow drivers each time I got in the car. I started yelling profanities at other drivers and pedestrians. According to Matt, it was like I was trying to pick a fight.

After encountering a dog off its leash in the backyard of our apartment complex one afternoon, I stormed back into the apartment.

"Matt, I'm fucking done with these idiots," I cried, slamming the door. "Nobody listens to the damn rules around here. Look, I got scratches all over my leg from saving the pups."

Walking out onto that balcony that overlooked the yard, I yelled, "You asshole, read the fucking sign. Put your dog on a leash. If this happens again, I'm kicking your ass."

Matt pulled me back in. "Knock it off Jason, you're making a scene!"

A few weeks later, I knocked back a few too many beers at the minor league baseball game. On our way out, I saw the neon green mosquito mascot standing there taking pictures with fans. As a mascot lover myself, I ran up to try and get a picture but apparently his shift was over. Enraged, I started cursing and shouting at the top of my lungs as we exited the stadium.

"Jason, stop," Matt said. "There are kids here. Everyone is looking at you." When we were finally in the car, Matt buried his head in his hands.

"I miss the positive person you were when we first met," Matt told me later that night.

But I was too busy to take it in, my mind more engrossed with the food we were eating.

CHAPTER 11

BODY MALFUNCTIONS

My childhood consisted of countless doctor visits. Ear infections, strep throat, you name it. I attributed this to my mom's late-in-life pregnancy, chain-smoking, and my own obesity. This was one of my motivating factors in maintaining my weight and eating healthy. I feared just one bad meal would cause weight gain and illness. I was sick of being sick.

Shortly before arriving in Texas, I noticed what appeared to be blood in my stool. I brushed it off, but I've always been a hypochondriac. You know the kind; you might even be one. You get a weird sensation in the big toe, and suddenly it's stage 4 cancer. This new symptom eventually haunted me enough to go to the doctor, who sent me for a colonoscopy "just to be safe."

The weekend leading up to the procedure felt like a horror movie with no end. I trembled with fear.

What would they find?

I frantically searched the Internet for diagnosis and survival rates.

Matt finally gave me something worth living for. How the hell could I die so young when my life was starting to look up?

I took the pups to the vet the day before my procedure and thought, *At least they'll have their vaccines before I die.* I figured the only bright side of the colonoscopy was the clearing out of my system and losing a couple of pounds in the process.

The doctor found three "very large polyps," which required a biopsy. He advised it could take up to ten days for the results. I tried to focus on my schoolwork, but anxiety paralyzed me. My unknown health status trapped me in a constant cycle of "what ifs". Every conversation I had with Matt somehow went back to the colonoscopy and the biopsy.

I kept picturing my dad's body vanishing before our eyes as cancer ate away at him. I relived the events preceding my dad's death: the way he yelped in pain while walking up the stairs, his yellowing skin, the way his hands grew thin and frail.

This would be my fate, too. I had always wanted to follow in his footsteps, but not like this. *Why couldn't this have happened before I met Matt and started a life together?* Love someone, and then death robs you of that.

Those weekend pizzas, or the nights out with friends, that's what caused it.

I researched every possible cause of colon cancer.

This is what you get for treating your body like a dumpster. Now, it's garbage day.

Chemotherapy, surgeries, and death invaded my mind before I even opened my eyes in the morning. My life felt like a video stuck on fast forward, with events coming up faster than expected. Then the call came: the results were in, but the doctor asked to meet in person to discuss what he saw. I called Matt at work, who rushed home to find a trembling wreck. My future hung in the balance as we headed to the doctor's office.

"I swear to God, if these results just come back negative, I will change my ways," I said, pulling at my face on the drive to the office. "I will eat as healthy as I can and take care of my body in any way possible. Just let me live."

To my enormous relief, the results were negative. But the news was not all good. According to the doctor, had I waited just a few more months, it might be a different story. I was now labeled as high-risk for colon cancer and would require yearly scopes. Yearly scopes at 29?! My polyps were the aggressive kind, my doctor explained. They sought total carnage.

I won this battle, but the war was just beginning. This life-changing event later served as the catalyst to my ultimate battle for survival. While I was relieved to have caught it in time, I was shell shocked that this was all happening before my 30th birthday. I blamed myself, my dad, and my genetics. I needed more control.

I have a fear of flying because I am not allowed in the cockpit. It does not matter if I may not understand the instruments or take over should something bad happen. My obsessive-compulsive nature needs to be in the know and take control. With the news of the polyps, I felt like my body had a mind of its own. It was like some sort of autopilot I couldn't switch off.

During my adolescence and early twenties, I dealt with more death and adult issues than my peers. Now, after a brief respite of feeling my age, here I was, dealing with colon polyps and cancer prospects. The VCR of my life appeared stuck on fast forward with my tape spinning out of control.

I had first heard the word "cancer" as a young child. My dad was talking with a friend at a diner about someone he knew who just lost a wife to the disease.

"What's cancer, Daddy?"

My dad gave me the PG version of it, but the thought of cancer sent chills down my spine. It sounded like a nasty case of strep throat or ear infection. I didn't understand what it was. I just knew I never wanted it. Some kids fear monsters at this age. Well, cancer was my boogie man lurking under the bed.

Thus, I was always on the lookout for cancer. The next scare came on a fall Saturday later that year while sitting on the couch watching my beloved Iowa Hawkeyes. I had reached for the clicker when I noticed that the brown eraser-sized spot on my elbow now appeared scaly with darker patches.

My eyes switched from the football game to the Internet. I frantically searched for pictures of melanoma, only to find website after website of horror stories. Several severe sunburns as a kid flashed before my eyes. Time to dust off the funeral arrangements again.

On Monday, I made the first available appointment with a dermatologist. He inspected the spot and assured me it was just a boring atypical mole—nothing to worry about.

Sweet Jesus. False Alarm!

I went about my normal business for several months until the mole caught my attention again. Now, it was itchy and starting to bleed. I visited a new dermatologist, who immediately decided the mole must be biopsied. He used a tool that reminded me of the hole punchers from grade school. One-click, and it was over. He bandaged the area up and said results would be back in a week or so.

Great, another week of torture and hell ahead.

My internet search history resembled that of an oncology student. I prepared for surgery, chemotherapy, and an early grave. Later that week, my doctor called with the results.

"Hi Jason, we've got good news and bad news," he said. His words cut through a beautiful spring day.

My heart stopped, "Okay what's going on?"

"Your mole has melanoma-like characteristics,"

Melanoma. Oh my God. Fuck! I'm dead.

"But fortunately, we caught it in time," he said. "It is not fully cancerous yet, but we will need to remove the entire area around the mole for safe margins."

My surgery was a success. There were no additional signs of melanoma and margins looked good. The twelve stitches on my arm and permanent scar served as remainders of my defective body.

I hate my poor health. I need more control.

I had hoped this was an isolated incident, but a few months later, we identified several other suspicious areas. All of these required painful removals, too. More stitches, more scars, and more fear of my own body.

It was almost no surprise to me at this point that my dermatologist declared me as high-risk for melanoma, which meant full-body checkups four times a year. I felt like my body, the only thing I truly owned, had it out for me. Orthorexia, unknown to me at the time, sat in the audience laughing. It plotted its next move as my relationship with food quickly deteriorated.

My sweet tooth was extracted when I discovered a couple websites that listed sugar as a cause of cancer. I also developed a phobia of red meat. Just looking at it in the display case of the grocery market made my insides tingle with fears of disease. I consumed websites and blogs that promoted healthy, preventive diets. Our pantry transformed into my own medicine cabinet, full of foods rich in vitamins and minerals thought to reduce the risk of cancer and disease. My relationship with food was not just for weight or body image any longer. My life now hung in the balance.

Maybe if I eat all organic produce and lots of it, I can prevent my next doctor's appointment from turning into my death row sentencing.

CHAPTER 12

GOOD VS. BAD

Hypochondriacs and natural worriers like myself use the Internet to self-diagnose in minutes. That stomach pain: cancer. This headache: stroke. It also enables a serial dieter to become their own dietitian.

Weight Watchers introduced me to nutrition basics, but that was the only formal diet I had ever followed. My quirky food regimens were solely based on personal interpretations.

The colon and skin biopsies changed that. I clearly needed more control to live. What I was doing might be keeping my weight down, but I now sought total health. I researched healthy alternatives to recipes I already loved. Sugar became enemy number one, FBI Most Wanted level because of studies suggesting a link to increased colorectal cancer risk.

Dr. Jason continued to search for foods to cut out in the name of health. While already leery of fats and carbohydrates, I started only seeing the bad in food, like how I only saw the bad in the world back then. I used social media influencers and fad diets I'd observe from others as my guide to "healthy eating."

One blogger seduced me with their Eat This, Not That! posts. She and her boyfriend had glowing skin in every picture. The vitamins and nutrients coursed from the perfect bodies and bright blond hair. His t-shirts stretched with bulging pecs and biceps. Her washboard abs seemed to scream *No cancer here. Join the fun!*

The couple encouraged diets like Whole30 and Keto. With that, I said goodbye to my good friends pasta and rice. I felt like I was back in high school, hearing the jeers and jabs about my body echoing across the locker room. I longed to live the life I believed everyone else had; lives in thin, muscular bodies that never had to deal with cancer. They were the antithesis to myself and my body that wanted to kill me. I had to control my food to survive the plane crash I was waiting to happen.

Maybe if I just cut out gluten, I can be healthier. And without sugar, I'm sure to avoid dying of cancer like my parents. Carbs are said to make you gain weight, which can cause diabetes, so I better stop that, too.

The list of bad foods grew exponentially. I inspected every nutrition label at the grocery store. I eventually stuck to the same "safe" items to prevent time-consuming investigation.

Eating out was no different. I despised restaurants that didn't provide nutritional information on their website. I treated a night out like a big test I needed to study for.

If the food was bad and I dared to eat it, then I was bad, too. One "bad" meal or snack equaled a boulder of guilt and shame on my back. Perhaps a part of me yearned for that remorse from food because it could numb the unresolved pain from years before. If I beat myself up about my diet, then I could forget about the hurt inside.

Alcohol provided a brief refuge from my pain and inner turmoil. It numbed the anger I felt for missing out on the college experience.

Even on my favorite days of the week watching college football, I often found myself fixated on the college campus and the kids in the crowd rather than the players on the field. This regret and loathing contributed to the heaping pile of empty beer bottles in the recycling bin every Saturday evening.

I continued to drink on the weekends, not unlike the way so many college kids consumed alcohol. In fact, come Friday or Saturday, I could easily knock back eight to ten beers a night. On special events like the Super Bowl or meeting up with friends, this number could exceed fifteen.

Intoxication made it easier to devour an entire cheesy pizza or a sizzling fajita platter, along with chips and salsa. Basket after basket, please.

"Wow, you're eating so late tonight. It's almost 9," Matt would say on a college football Saturday.

"Yeah, it's bad luck to eat before the game is over," was my typical excuse.

I needed to be drunk to treat myself. Granted, the remorse punched sober Jason in the mouth the next morning, I was only happy when I was drunk. I lived for the weekends when I could drink and eat freely. The man of the house does not show jealousy or hurt, and drinking helped to cover up all of that. I continued to only show the Jason who lost all the weight in high school, and the resilient man who could handle the death of both parents. There was no playing victim here—only toughness.

This tough Jason fooled the grieving, terrified Jason beneath.

CHAPTER 13

AN ENGAGING MOMENT

In 2018, Matt booked a European adventure to celebrate my college graduation. This was my first time across the pond. A whole new world! Granted, I spent most of the time anticipating where we would eat to plan accordingly. This meant I found places with "safe" foods and insisted we eat there several times during our stay. There was no leaving my comfort zone, even on a different continent. The eating disorder must have purchased a seat on our flight over there.

I've always loved black forest cherry cake, and I swore that I would have to get some while in Europe. A quaint little cafe in Potsdam, Germany, had it on the menu.

Potsdam is a short train ride from the urban bustle of Berlin. The historic city combines architecture with nature to create a dreamlike aura—a place where kings once stayed. Matt and I sat under a blue umbrella as raindrops splashed on the cobblestones. I looked forward to this moment throughout the trip.

Then panic set in when the server placed the cake in front of me. I felt guilty before I even committed the crime. I wanted to back out, but I knew I couldn't. Matt would be upset that I dragged him to this cafe in the rain. I watched him nibble on some fries while I quietly judged the greasy snack in my head. I finally found the courage to dig in. It was delicious. It had the perfect balance of bitter chocolate and sour cherry. I ate the whole slice.

As each spongy bite went down, my attention drifted to a table of young men sitting across from us. Their bodies had the perfect amount of muscle to fill out their t-shirts but not to the extent of a Jersey Shore cast member. Not more than thirty, they seemed the epitome of perfect health. They were like the bloggers I read online.

I'd already observed the men polish off a beer with brunch, and then order dessert around the same time I ordered my cake. The anger, frustration, and lack of self-respect started boiling up within me. As the guys laughed together, I wondered how they could have this much fun even with their greasy, fatty food. How the hell did they stay in shape like that? If I ate like them, I'd gain twenty pounds in one sitting and probably develop diabetes. My mind was no longer on the cake in front of me. It was no longer on Matt and this historic avenue. I wanted to be like those guys. The same feelings rushed over me from the high school locker room.

Why did I get stuck with a body that doesn't look and behave like everyone else's?

After the meal, Matt and I headed to Prague, "the City of a Hundred Spires," for the second leg of the trip. Hugged by the Vltava River, this fairytale town was made up of perfectly preserved gothic and medieval architecture. Castles and cathedrals dotted the landscape, cobblestone streets flooded with laughter, and historic bridges arched across the river's flowing waters. The forecast called for rain our first evening there. In typical Jason fashion, I went to work identifying indoor options for entertainment.

Vacations are usually planned down to the minute. As a kid, I prepared a detailed weekend agenda for our family vacations to the Wisconsin Dells. My obsessive-compulsive disorder and anxiety often require everything to be planned as far in advance as possible. This only grew as an adult. If I couldn't control my painful past, at least I still had a chance at the future.

A riverboat dinner cruise appeared to be the perfect rainy night option. Matt loved the idea, and we booked our tickets. I wore a button-down shirt with a collar that night, the sign of a special occasion.

The single-level boat looked like a glass pill capsule. A friendly hostess, wearing traditional black and white attire, greeted us with a tray of Prosecco.

"Can you believe this? I feel so VIP," I said to Matt as we sat at a table for two next to the glass exterior of the boat.

Dry from the storm, Matt and I enjoyed the buffet dinner and entertainment while taking in the glow from the city lights on the flowing river. The champagne washed away the worries of food that evening. This was a new level of romance for me and the tall, dark, handsome man across the table.

Matt and I headed to a little bar following the cruise. Jazz music erupted from the downstairs venue while lightning lit up the wet cobblestone outside. Caught up in the magic of the evening, my mind was free of stress and anxiety. It was a brief refuge from the storm.

As the two of us splashed through the uneven streets towards our rental that night, Matt said that he wanted to stop and check out the Charles Bridge. I couldn't understand why since we walked over that historic bridge several times throughout the day.

When we reached the bridge, I stood, admiring the brute force of nature and the history surrounding me. The city lights reflected off the dark river and lightning illuminated the church steeples and clock towers. "Turn around, look at this," Matt said. When I rotated toward him, I found Matt down one knee. The ring box had an LED light in it that lit up the tears welling up in Matt's eyes. "Will you marry me?"

I'd been waiting nearly eight years for this moment. Matt really wanted me to be his husband.

Wow, I am worthy of love. And whoa, could this be any more romantic?

I couldn't speak at first. I wanted to cherish this moment of love without messing it up. I finally exclaimed, "Yes, yes!" As we embraced, I thought, I will finally have an immediate family, an intimate connection since the last time I held my mom's hand.

∾

When I got up the next morning, I was ready to start planning. Matt reminded me that we should focus on the rest of the trip. "We can plan stateside," he said. "We'll be home next week."

Okay, fair point.

Reality seeped in during breakfast. This wedding represented my first opportunity to show family members and friends how far I'd come from my late teens and early twenties. I had to be in shape to impress them and act like I had a perfect life. This was the equivalent of my Miss America pageant. My Oscars. My Super Bowl.

The cafe buzzed with life, espresso, and European pastries. Our cozy table exploded with plates of French toast covered with blackberries, strawberries, and blueberries; flaky, golden croissants; and savory, shiny omelets. The combination of maple syrup, powdered sugar, and fruit awoke my taste buds and the inner judge in my head.

Okay, you can have this one celebratory meal. But after this, no more treats. You must be perfect for your wedding, and as healthy as possible. Do you really want to leave Matt a widower at a young age?

A few days later, we found ourselves at a picturesque cafe nestled in a cozy, residential neighborhood of Berlin. Matt ordered a golden-brown croissant that oozed with butter. The fresh preserves on the side looked like the perfect balance of tart and sweet. I wanted one, too. In fact, most people at the cafe enjoyed a croissant with their breakfast. However, I had a wedding to prepare for and had already treated myself too much during the trip.

"I've eaten so many croissants already," I said. "Let me try something new." This was my excuse for my measly scrambled egg whites and fruit bowl. I still think about that Berlin cafe and how much I wish I had actually ordered what I wanted.

CHAPTER 14

WEIGHTY EXPECTATIONS

I crafted a twenty-three-tab spreadsheet for the wedding plan the same week we returned home to Houston. We set a date for later the following year, which meant I didn't have to get super strict with my diet just yet. I continued with my normal food regimen of strict weekdays and lax weekends.

However, my body was changing. Life never slows down, but metabolism sure does. Five or six times a day, I found myself heading to the bathroom for my regular appointment with the scale.

The typical week looked like an inverted bell curve. Monday started out heaviest due to the weekend binges. I often attributed water weight from alcohol and sodium as the cause.

I felt disgusting, instantly regretting the freedom of the weekend. I dreaded the thought of putting on work clothes Monday morning, more so than the work itself. Pants fit tighter and shirts showed every curve. It was not out of the norm to try on several different outfits before I found the perfect mask for my weekend binges. If things went right and I followed my strict regimen, I returned to my lowest weight by Thursday evening or Friday morning before climbing back up over the weekend.

Holidays and special events always threw a wrench in my plans, as did dinner out with friends during the week. These events made it difficult to reach my weight goals by the end of the workweek.

"Hey, Elizabeth invited us out to La Tapatia tonight," Matt texted me one morning.

Matt's message stoked panic within.

What will I order? This was not planned. Why would they just ask us out of the blue?

I arrived at the lively Mexican restaurant that evening to find our friends surrounded by margaritas, chips, salsa, queso and guacamole. While the mariachi music and laughter of friends sounded inviting, I would have rather been going to the dentist.

"Um, I'll have two chicken tacos and a skinny margarita, please," I said. I hoped the waitress couldn't hear the hesitation in my voice. I really wanted enchiladas, but they seemed like cancer time bombs drenched in sauce and cheese.

"They have the best chips and salsa in town," someone at the table remarked, grabbing a crispy, salty chip and dunking it in the rainbow of dips.

Maybe I could eat just one. Could I have just one?

No. You did not plan for this. Just eat your tacos and shut up.

We were developing closer friendships with Matt's co-workers, our first true friends since moving to Houston. This posed a threat to the control I had over my diet. Invitations out for dinner were now becoming more frequent. So I started brainstorming a list of excuses to decline these last-minute curveballs. I wanted to see and meet friends, but I felt like I couldn't even concentrate on the conversation with the food police barking in my ear.

While my strategy of strict weekdays and free-for-all weekends proved effective during my twenties, I found the thirties were not as kind. My high-end numbers on Monday reached new highs and my low-end numbers on Friday morning failed to meet my expectations. I could no longer do the one thing I was good at. Even worse, the heavy feeling I usually felt on Mondays now plagued me all week.

My mind told me I was opening the door to disease, cancer, and failure. I panicked. The fears of once again being different because of my weight flooded my mind. With the holidays approaching, I prepared myself for the typical five-to-ten-pound weight gain. What can I say? I love pumpkin beer and Christmas cookies. I always felt shame and remorse on New Year's Day, but I came to expect this, and I knew the tools to lose weight.

Time to get strict again. So long dessert.

Now, where are those hunger pains to tell me I'm a success?

Nine months from the wedding, morning visits to the scale revealed my heaviest weight in ten years. This holiday weight gain was more than ever before. My current meal plan was no longer effective. My weekends consisted of binge after binge. Four slices of meatloaf, cheddar bay biscuits, mashed potatoes, and cookies washed down with a dozen beers became the typical Sunday night feast. Then it was right back to work Monday morning, but five days were no longer enough to get to my goal weight.

Yo-yo weight trends turned into a single "yo."

Yo, you need to stop eating so much and get it together.

Matt surprised me with a New Year's trip to Tampa Bay. The Iowa Hawkeyes were playing in the Outback Bowl. Since it was the middle of winter and a total surprise trip, I was not prepared to show off the holiday bod or blob as I would refer to it back then. As I packed, I tried on one pair of shorts that no longer fit. Then another, and another.

You fat pig, look at yourself. What have you done? Failure.

Matt and I decided to head to Tampa's outlet mall for some new shorts and a New Year's Eve outfit. I loved the clothes on the rack but hated them on me. Guilt, remorse, shame, and embarrassment overwhelmed that tiny J-Crew changing room. The jiggly man in the mirror repulsed me while the voices of high school bullies echoed in my head.

Later that day, I wore a black t-shirt to Clearwater Beach to cover up as much as possible. Black is slimming, right? It was nearly 85 degrees, and I was surrounded by guys who felt comfortable enough to take their shirts off. Their muscular and toned bodies screamed success compared to my flabby failure. It didn't help that most of the beachgoers were collegiate athletes, cheerleaders, and football players. At one point, Matt joined the shirtless crowd.

"Oh my God, what are you doing? You're taking your shirt off?" I exclaimed like it was some sort of felony to show a little skin.

"Well yeah, we're at the beach. What are you wearing? You look like Morticia Addams," he replied with a chuckle.

"I don't want to get burnt," I lied.

During the drive home from Tampa, I vowed to book a personal trainer immediately. This was my time to be like the muscular jocks we saw on Clearwater Beach. My friends would no longer poke fun at my toothpick arms because I was going to get shredded.

Can you imagine the looks on my friends' and relatives' faces when they see muscular Jason walk down the aisle in September?

That will show them how far I've come.

CHAPTER 15

THE WEDDING DIET

An American Gladiator stood before me one week later in the gym—my new personal trainer, Austin. As tough as this guy looked with his bulging biceps, he had the personality of the boy next door. Austin built clients up instead of barking commands at them. I knew if someone could help me achieve my goal of total health with a gentle spirit, this would be the guy.

"I want to lose this excess fat I gained over the past year and replace it with muscle," I explained. "I'm getting married later this year and want to wow my friends and family."

"Let's get it done, man," Austin said. "Between working out and tracking your food intake, it'll happen."

Austin told me I would need to increase my protein and calorie intake over time to build muscle. This concept seemed counterintuitive to my one-track mind.

I want to lose this fat and be healthy and he's telling me I'll need to eat more?

I decided to listen to Austin in the gym, but my nutrition tracking log was a different story. I fudged my numbers much like I did in

Weight Watchers. After all, I knew how to overachieve, and I was going to lose this weight my way.

Austin recommended a fitness app for us to track my diet and exercise. I religiously updated the app throughout the day, but I cooked the books. The perfect student inside strove for praise and attention. I wanted my fat gone there and now. I had a wedding coming up and a life to live for.

I also returned to my beloved fitness and diet blogs, which portrayed carbohydrates as an unnecessary evil. I bookmarked a chart that ranked foods on the Glycemic Index. This quickly became my precedent for what carbohydrates made the cut. Website after website and influencer after influencer raved about diets like Keto and Paleo as if they were magical remedies.

A former co-worker tried Adkins and cut out all carbs. He lost weight but seemed miserable in the process. Another co-worker wound up in the hospital after taking on Whole30.

While I liked the basis of these diets, I figured I could modify them to stay safe. I limited my carbohydrates to whole grains and fruits in the morning. Then lunch and dinner were predominantly protein. After all, protein equals muscle, according to all the gym rats online. I divorced several beloved foods like peanut butter because of the fat content and fruits like pineapple, which contained too much sugar according to the Keto blogs online.

Macros became my new buzzword since it was all about loading up on protein and watching carbs and fat. I also reduced my drinking to a few glasses of wine on the weekend and stopped the weekend binges. Every day became a workday, with no time off. Perfect body, perfect health, perfect me.

Just like my first endeavor into dieting, the pounds vanished in no time.

"Wow, man, you look incredible," Austin said a couple months after working with him. You're making fast progress. Can I feature you in a client update post on Facebook? I'm so proud of all you've accomplished."

I dropped almost twenty pounds in six weeks. As my body shrank, my confidence grew. I figured I was well on my way to that dream beach body now.

CHAPTER 16

PRIDE AND PREJUDICE

Next up on the wedding spreadsheet: find a suit. This was going to be a difficult task for a basketball shorts and ratty t-shirt kind of guy. The wedding, however, ignited my inner Vogue. I set out on a mission to find the perfect suit for the perfect day—the suit to cling to my new figure and show off my accomplishments.

Brides get to pick out their wedding dress to much fanfare, as do gay guys with their suits. The initial visit was just the fitting, but I dreaded it. I didn't want a stranger to measure every nook and cranny and find all my imperfections. That was why I stuck to my basketball shorts.

The stylist greeted me at the door. His skinny suit revealed a perfectly toned body. He was the ideal walking mannequin for a high-end men's suit store.

Damn, I wish I could wear skinny clothes like that.

"Okay Mr. Wood, let me get your measurements."

"Just a heads up, I know I have thick legs," I said with a laugh to lighten my embarrassment.

"Well, your waist seems in line with our standard size guide. Why don't you try these on?" He handed me a couple suit combinations.

Inside the fitting room, I found myself tugging at the first pair of pants to get the itchy fabric over my calves. One foot in, then the next foot, now pull up.

Within a moment, I knew I needed the jaws of life to get me out of those suckers

Fatass, disappointment, embarrassment.

"Um . . . excuse me," I said, peeking out of the curtain. "Could we try another size? These seem to be tight in the legs."

The stylist brought over another cut of the pants, which again choked off at my knees.

"Do you have a larger size?" I asked, feeling the heat rise in my face.

"Well, we do, but unfortunately, it will be way too large around the waist. I'm sorry, sir, but we'll probably need to go the custom route with you since our suits are sold in sets. I'll get the custom paperwork for you to review at home."

I fought back tears while looking at the half-clothed creature staring back at me in the full-length mirror. His upper half was perfectly shaped by the slim suit jacket, while the bottom half rejected the pants that matched. It looked like somebody had copy and pasted another person's legs on my skinny frame.

I detested shopping for pants ever since the husky days of childhood. While I lost a substantial amount of weight in high school, my calves never seemed to follow suit with the rest of my body. Friends complimented my calves since a lot of fitness fanatics strive for calves the size of mine, but all I could see was how disproportionate they were to the rest of my body.

Skinny jeans had always been out of the question. And when I tried on suits in this moment for the wedding, all I could see was baggy in the butt, skin-tight on the calf. Style and cut didn't seem to make a difference. Styles always looked perfect on the rack until my calves got their say. Just like my husky jeans in elementary school and gym uniform in high school, my fat calves required a custom-made suit. It was a heavy price tag and burden to bear.

The scale provided me with numbers I liked. The stylist's tape measure did not. The hate for my calves grew while my determination to make them disappear raged.

"Austin, what can we do to make my legs smaller?" I asked my personal trainer.

"Well bro, we can tone them up, but you're just one of the lucky guys with big calves. Much better than those guys who have big chests and tiny legs. We'll work on tightening them up for you."

Damn, I'm stuck with these monsters. Toning won't be enough.

I increased my cardio sessions in search of the magical formula to reduce the size of my calves. Thirty minutes of cardio now became sixty, if not ninety minutes.

~

At work, social gatherings like potlucks were my definition of hell. And this is coming from someone who is now an office events coordinator.

I used to love potlucks and work get-togethers, but my unhealthy relationship with food made me a recluse at work. I needed to know the ingredients in each dish. I didn't trust the people around me, judging them solely on what they ate.

I snuck out most of the days that I knew a potluck was happening to avoid having to come up with an excuse. I even missed out on the office-wide Thanksgiving lunch by scheduling a call at the same time.

My headset failed to block out the laughter coming from the long folding tables where my co-workers feasted.

I feared their fatty foods high in sugar and salt. I stuck to my "safe" Chipotle salad bowl: no rice, just lettuce, veggies, black beans, chicken, and one salsa. No way could I have two salsas thanks to the sodium.

I often hosted guests at our office, which meant catering breakfast and lunch. Breakfast was easy because I woke up early and used the excuse that I already ate. Lunch proved much more challenging. On one occasion, my visitors chowed down on pasta and sandwiches while I sat in the six-person meeting room with my half of a leftover Chipotle salad bowl.

"Why don't you have some of this pasta, Jason? It's incredible," remarked one of my close friends from a visiting firm. She seemed so carefree as those evil carbohydrates entered her mouth.

"Well, I'm on my wedding diet," I said with pride. "I started working with a personal trainer and reduced my carb intake. I haven't cut all carbs because that seems too extreme."

My fellow lunchmates nodded in agreement. "Yeah, I should really cut back too but I just love pasta and bread too much," joked one guy. The room erupted in agreeing giggles.

"Haha, yeah. It's funny, I don't even miss carbs now," I lied. "Plus, I've already lost twenty pounds and feel great. Now I'm just focused on eating a lot of protein to build muscle. I don't want to lose any more weight."

"Wow, that's incredible," several guests remarked.

"Your willpower is impressive. I couldn't do that."

Others nodded in agreement as they continued to slurp down their spaghetti. Suddenly, I didn't feel so bad crunching down another piece of iceberg lettuce covered in bean juice.

Another morning, my neighboring co-worker arrived clutching two white boxes from Shipley Donut. I eyed the grease-painted corners of the paper container as the woman carrying the box invited me to grab a donut. Co-workers jumped from their seats to grab the sugary delights while I scooped away at my chia seed pudding and kiwi.

Look at those wild savage pigs, ready to devour anything in sight. They don't love themselves or their bodies as much as I do. Look at my amazing willpower.

I used to be a Homer Simpson for doughnuts. Those days felt like lightyears ago. Now, I was sure the sugar would feed cancer that lurked somewhere in my body.

And I'll never forget the morning my busybody coworker talked about the benefits of drinking green tea every day to boost your metabolism and cleanse the body. I watched as fellow office mates hung on her every word.

Blasphemy. How dare she say this after I just watched her eat a sandwich and doughnut the other day.

I was the one who drank green tea every morning for those benefits. I judged my coworker as a false prophet for the remainder of my days at the company.

But work wasn't the only place where I could show off my willpower and discipline. Buffalo Wild Wings, at one time my favorite chain sports bar, became the next location where I had to make new food choices thanks to my diet.

Every year during the opening round of March Madness, you could find me at a table near the bar with my bracket in one hand, beer in another, and my eyes fixed on the games. I easily spent all day there.

This year, my go-to grilled chicken wrap with Asian zing found itself on the naughty list. Studying the nutrition facts before my next visit, a part of me died when I saw the sodium count and grams of sugar in my beloved Asian zing sauce. With my favorite menu item blacklisted, I immediately analyzed the nutrition menu like a forensics scientist. Too many carbs there, too much fat here. It seemed everything on the menu belonged in food jail.

I finally settled on their soft-shell tacos. I could scrape off the shredded cheese and only eat the protein-dense filling. This meant no tortilla shell, which basically left some chunks of grilled chicken, lettuce, and pico de gallo on my plate. My calculations deemed spicy garlic a suitable sauce selection; however, it would have to be on the side. This way, I could limit my sodium count.

The big day arrived without the same anticipation of past years. The morning was spent fearing how many calories and what type of macros I would consume. And for twelve hours at Buffalo Wild Wings, my focus drifted from the games to the plates of food coming out around me.

I peered at a couple sharing chips and salsa as an appetizer. I hated myself more with each crunch of the chips. Then, a young lady at the bar ordered a large plate of wings for her lunch. She didn't seem to care about the nutrition or the messy sauce, yet her body was toned, and she looked as if she was just leaving her daily spin class. Had I seen her without the plate of bones in front of her, I'd think she was the epitome of perfect health.

What kind of sick individual has a large order of wings for lunch slathered in fat and salt?

I dissected my two little tacos, arrogantly picking out the chicken chunks and lettuce. Then I'd gently dip each forkful into the sauce.

I wanted to announce to the entire restaurant that I was better than them.

I mean, just look at my amazing willpower.

Lunch was subpar. Let's just say you don't go to Buffalo Wild Wings for tacos. Whatever. I had pleased the inner judge in my head. I could spend the rest of the afternoon free of the guilt that would have waltzed into my life with one chip or dip of Asian zing.

Matt arrived in time for dinner. "Should I get the medium or large order of wings?" he asked, grabbing a seat at the bar.

"Well, you do love your wings. Why don't you go for the large?" I suggested.

Meanwhile, I ordered small wings with dry rub seasoning. The dry rub seemed like the fountain of youth due to the low nutritional count. I justified the wings as a source of protein.

We also ordered a pretzel to share. And when I say share, I mean I ate one or two bites and let Matt have the rest.

Here Matt goes on his gluttonous ways.

Man, I have some amazing willpower. Everyone else is just so weak.

How could I think this about the man I loved, the man I planned to marry in six months?

"Oh wow, I think I ate too much." Matt declared victory to his chicken counterparts.

Yes, yes, yes! The voice in my head sounded like a villain hatching another evil plot. A part of me found pleasure in his regret because it further proved how good I was at healthy eating. This became a regular occurrence over the coming weeks and months as my illness took hold.

I left Buffalo Wild Wings that night an empty winner. My bracket survived, my diet survived, but my morale did not. I missed the so-called "bad" foods, but I believed that this had to be my new normal. This was what I had to do to prevent dying young and impress everyone around me.

CHAPTER 17

THE BACHELOR PARTY

My bachelor party back in Illinois represented an opportunity to catch up with close friends; however, it also signaled another excursion outside the comfort zone of strict meal and workout regimens. My overnight oats in the morning would not be there. Dinner would be out with friends. And the alcohol, well, this was my drinking crew, so I better prepare for all those extra calories.

I should have been thrilled to see my friends and celebrate my pending nuptials, yet I approached the trip with caution. In a reversal from the Tampa trip, many of my clothes were now too big. I was eager to show off my accomplishments but dreaded the temptations to go off track.

My first stop was the Chicago institution known as Portillo's. I swear the grease from their hot dogs, sausages and crinkle-cut fries flows through every Chicagoan's veins. If they could turn the savory smells of that restaurant into a candle, I'd buy a hundred.

My mom and I ate a lot of Portillo's back in the day. I'd order a big beef, large cheese fry and wash it down with a slice of chocolate cake. We'd catch up on life and shout out answers while watching her favorite game shows. In preparation for Portillo's, I refrained from eating most of the day. I even cut back on my staple Chipotle salad bowl: no beans, just to be safe. I saved the calories and carbs for dinner.

Before heading to my friend's house, I hit up the drive thru. Wood, party of one. The smell of French fries and grease floated through the car window as I asked for a regular Italian beef with hot and sweet peppers. If I skipped the cheese and the big size beef, then I would not completely kill myself with this meal.

Afraid of appearing weak in front of friends, I sat at the edge of the parking lot to eat dinner alone. I unwrapped the beef sandwich. The Italian hoagie bread, cradling thinly sliced beef, dripped with au jus and shimmered in a thin glaze of fat. One deep breath, and in I went. The juice from the beef drizzled down my chin. Wow, it tasted incredible. Just one bite took me back to childhood, to happier times.

But I couldn't outrun the feeling that I was committing some heinous act. This beef would surely cause multiple polyps during my next colonoscopy. My chest tightened, simulating the heart attack I anticipated from the sodium and fat. It seemed as if my belly popped right back out for the first time in months. Four months of hard work vanished with one bite.

I managed to eat a few more bites, but the joy died quickly. It was akin to the feeling you get on December 26 when Christmas is over, and you didn't get what you wanted. I started questioning why the hell I ordered a small fry on top of it all. Their crinkle-cut fries with the perfect crisp outside and piping hot silky smooth inside used to be heaven in a bite. Today, they were a sin. That sack of fries represented my failure at sticking to the plan.

That damn smell when I rolled down my window to order must have seduced me.

I hastily wrapped up what was left of the beef sandwich and threw it back in the red and white striped bag along with a full sack of fries. I found the closest garbage can and tossed the evidence in the trash.

There would be no drinking for me tonight. My body reached its max for the day, with no more calories in. I grabbed a large decaf coffee before heading to my friends.

They're not going to expect you to have a beer when you're mid-coffee.

I worried that my friends wouldn't see the hard work I had put in on the wedding diet. But as expected, they did just that.

"Wow, you look great," one said.

"Oh, you're so skinny!" exclaimed another.

I lived for these comments. It justified my diet plan. I finally had the body everybody wanted. Childhood shame became adulthood pride.

The day of my bachelor party was also Kentucky Derby Day. We planned a big celebration at my home track, which would also serve as my wedding venue later that year.

"What are you doing for breakfast?" asked one friend.

"Want to grab doughnuts in the morning?" asked another.

I cut off any temptation with a quick. "Would love to, but I already promised a friend I'd do breakfast with them."

Of course, there was no friend to meet that next morning. Instead, I had an appointment with Starbucks, where I could order several menu items on my safe list before the booze flowed later in the day.

My friends and I had an amazing time at the track, and thanks to the unprecedented disqualification of Maximum Security, I won several hundred dollars on the race. Oh, and I ate a hot dog, bun and all. Alcohol and horse racing quieted the voices in my head long enough to live in the moment and celebrate with my friends. It was a brief respite from the growing storm within.

At dinner, I watched my friends order exactly what they wanted. Everyone laughed and ate. Our long table mimicked that of The Last Supper, except we were a bunch of tipsy millennials in big hats and bowties. My pre-trip reconnaissance led to a shrimp bowl with cauliflower rice. I didn't really want to eat that with so many other appetizing options on the menu, but I forced myself to order it anyway. My caloric intake for the day was already shot to hell thanks to mint juleps and beer.

My friend's suggestion for a couple appetizers was met with a round of "yeahs" by the table. I refrained from voting, much like I refrained from partaking in any of the appetizers. Of course, they placed the nachos down right in front of me.

Nope, not happening, Jason. You've treated yourself too much this trip and have to look strong in front of your posse.

The dim lighting at the restaurant couldn't hide the meager amount of food on my plate in comparison to my friends' burgers, chicken strips, and creamy pasta bowls. The shrimp bowl was fresh, but it lacked much in the way of spice or flare. The cauliflower rice pooled at the bottom of the bowl in its boring slimy way. My blackberry bourbon cocktail helped fill some of the empty feeling inside.

The bachelor party antics continued when a small group of us decided to hit up my favorite bar. The beer flowed as the clock ticked away the night. Other patrons slowly stumbled their way out the door. The four of us stayed, laughing and reminiscing about days gone by.

After several hours, we loaded into an Uber for the short trip back to my friend's house. On the way, we passed our group's go-to late-night Mexican joint. It was a little hole-in-the-wall restaurant, open until three in the morning. Their burritos tasted like garbage come daylight, but they were as good as a filet mignon with lobster tail at this hour.

"We have to stop," I declared.

The driver obliged and assisted our drunk asses in getting that late-night Mexican fix, which is about the last thing I remember from the night. Alcohol got the last swing, and I was down for the count. I woke up the next morning with a headache of guilt and remorse. I was at the mercy of a binge regret hangover. I saw the empty bag of chips and salsa next to the greased stained brown bag that once housed a silver-wrapped burrito.

Oh no, what did I do?

I wanted to punch that guilty face in the mirror. That late-night pit stop was not on my food agenda. My weeks of preparation crumbled with each dip of the fried tortilla into the bowl of spicy salsa.

Alcohol enabled me to eat that garbage. I would have never done that if I was sober. Jeez, Jason, can't you do anything right?

Worst of all, I knew my friends witnessed the crime. How could they have one ounce of respect when they saw me eat all the stuff I preached against earlier in the day? I certainly lost all respect for myself.

That morning I hopped in my car and drove about an hour out of town to DeKalb, a small college town that divided the endless cornfields. It was an area I commonly went to reflect on life when I lived in Illinois. Not only was it a quiet oasis, but it also made me feel like a college student, which placed a bandage over the scars from missing out on the college experience myself. Pulling over to the side of the road, I began to cry.

You suck at the one thing you think you're good at. This is why you always have bad things happen to you. Your past is a result of your constant failures.

I vowed to be even stricter with my diet. Alcohol had to be eliminated because it enabled this binge of forbidden foods. I needed to get back home to Houston, where I could resume my research of the healthiest diets. I also committed to working out seven days a week. I didn't deserve a rest day unless I wanted to be fat at my wedding and then die at a young age like my parents. Hell, at this point, I was already half the age my dad was when he died.

Relief and remorse flowed over my body as I boarded the plane Monday morning. I sat down in my seat, buckled up, and pressed my head on the cold window. My fast-blinking eyelids kept the tears of defeat dammed up inside.

CHAPTER 18

LEAN AND GREEN

A work trip to Greenville, South Carolina, loomed on the horizon. I would be there all week to host a conference, and then Matt planned to meet me for Memorial Day weekend in Charleston. We dreamed of visiting the historic coastal town for years and jumped at the opportunity to do so.

Matt's level of anticipation for the trip matched mine of internal dread. Eight days away from home meant no personal trainer, eating out for every meal, and being away from my rigid routine. Co-workers would expect me to grab a drink with them, while the wonderful restaurants of Greenville would tempt me with their southern charm and hospitality.

Previous trips to Greenville consisted of BBQ, fried pickles, and beer. I used to be able to visit and treat myself to a working vacation. This time, however, I felt like I was headed off to war.

I brainstormed a list of excuses to get out of social gatherings with co-workers and friends. Meetings at lunchtime became one of my go-to excuses, as did being tired from the flight. I even lied about what day I arrived to avoid dinner with one of our vendors. My flight got in early Sunday, but I told them I wouldn't be in until early Monday.

As usual, I spent days researching restaurant menus. My favorite places from previous trips were off the list. The sports bars with their fried foods represented hurdles to my strict diet. I identified a counter-service style joint that specialized in salad and grain bowls. If I stayed away from the cream-based cilantro-lime dressing, I'd be okay.

After dropping off the luggage at the hotel, I was off to the grocery store to stock up on low-fat yogurts and fruits. And by 5am the next morning, I was off to the workout room.

The hotel elevator rattled its way down to the main level where the doors parted to reveal a quaint hotel gym. Fear sparked within me as soon as I heard the buzz of a treadmill.

Fuck.

I opened the door to the gym and turned to my left where I saw two women occupying the only two treadmills. This had never happened in my previous stays here.

How did they get up earlier than me?

The rain outside and an early meeting meant this guy was not getting his cardio in. This was not in my workout plan. Control lost. I retreated to my room, where I proceeded to have a panic attack. My heart slammed against my rib cage and my palms moistened with sweat.

After several minutes of deep breathing, I collected myself and determined I could still do weight training that day. I returned to the gym and lifted; however, this gym didn't have the equipment I was used to. I missed my personal trainer to help guide me. And my muscles lacked the typical burn from a good workout.

The rest of my day was ruined by the time the sun rose over upstate South Carolina. All it took was one subpar workout—something not going according to plan, and I was down for the count. Yet, I still had to don the mask of cheerfulness and fake excitement. Acting upbeat and positive around my co-workers required a lot of energy. The people in the Greenville office were always so friendly and interested in my life. "How's the wedding planning coming along? You look incredible." Their true southern hospitality shone through. I forced a smile and went to work doing the other thing I excelled at: putting on a character.

"Yeah, I reduced my carb intake and started working with a personal trainer. I've never felt better," I said. My persuasion skills were so good I could often fool myself into believing I was thrilled no matter how miserable I felt.

Several of the visitors who joined me for lunch in Houston were also in Greenville. When they arrived, I ran up, gave them a hug, and welcomed them to the conference I was in town to host. One of my favorite ladies stepped back, hand covering her mouth. "Oh my god, honey, you are getting way too thin. We need to fatten you up this week."

Her words hit like a hurricane. One part of me beamed with glee as she justified my hard work. This is the reaction I wanted but also the one I hated. Yes, I loved being called thin. Who wouldn't when you were called "Fatty" and "Porkchop" during your childhood? But I also despised people inserting their noses into my weird eating habits.

"I'm not even trying to lose any more weight," I said. "Don't worry. I'm just eating healthy and putting on muscle for the wedding."

"Well, please be safe and take care of yourself. You already look great."

I felt like Stretch Armstrong with my ego pulling me in one direction and my anger pulling me in another. *Too skinny?!* I couldn't see it. I had a personal trainer, I still ate food, and I wasn't purging.

I was eating healthy and taking care of myself. High school health class never classified those desires as unhealthy.

I don't know what she's worried about. They're all just jealous that they can't put in the level of dedication I can.

On Thursday, I sat on the outdoor patio of the hotel eagerly awaiting Matt's arrival. I pre-selected the restaurant to ensure dinner would meet my health standards. A plate of cooked vegetables and a filet of salmon with no sauce awaited me. My strategic planning ensured a fun night free of food anxiety or self-regret.

Matt and I strolled down the main street amid the glow of restaurants and bars. The river flowed over the rapids and echoed through the trees. This night seemed perfect until Matt got the craving for some ice cream.

Oh no. No, no, no. This is not on the agenda.

Matt pointed to a bright store front filled with customers. It was the kind of ice cream shop where they pour the liquid cream onto a cold marble surface, and it freezes into a thin layer. Then they use a flat-blade utensil, similar to an ice scraper for a car's windshield, to roll up the ice cream before mixing in the toppings. Matt, thirty-five at the time, morphed into a ten-year-old boy before my eyes. I've always loved that about him. But at that moment, I felt like a deer in headlights.

We used to eat ice cream together all the time. Matt and I would gather the pups in the car, drive to an ice cream shop, and kick back a waffle cone while the pups licked away at their own sundaes. Those summer evenings felt like a different lifetime now. Yeah, the fear of gaining weight accompanied me on those outings, but I could still silence the guilt and shame long enough to enjoy my cone. Ever since the cancer scare, however, I could not get past the fear of impending doom.

"Oh, we should stop here before we get back to the room," Matt exclaimed.

"Oh, okay, sure, this looks fun," I said, forcing a smile.

We stood in line for ten minutes watching creamy creation after creation come to life. Laughter, love, and the seducing smell of fresh waffle cones filled the lively parlor. Everyone seemed so happy. Everyone but me.

I analyzed the menu. Their extensive collection of toppings ranged from fresh berries to Heath Bar crumbles and gummy worms. I checked my fitness tracking app, praying I could find enough calories to eat just the smallest ice cream sundae. The app replied with a sound NO! I reached my macros and couldn't have anything else.

"Oh man, I'm stuffed from dinner. Maybe I'll have a bite of yours," I said.

Matt shrugged, seemingly satisfied with my response. Salvation from that shame-inducing ice cream treat.

Matt gobbled down his ice cream. Oh, how bad I wanted to enjoy this dessert, too. Instead, I focused on judging everybody else. It didn't matter if the ice cream-eater was in the best shape of their life or overweight; they all seemed like weaklings to me.

Matt and I departed for Charleston the next morning. My anxiety heightened with the temptations that lay ahead. Would I drink too much and binge again? Is Matt going to throw another surprise dessert my way? Where is the healthiest restaurant I can eat each meal?

I spent most of the car ride researching the healthiest places to eat. Matt and I talked about plans for the wedding, but my mind was elsewhere. I needed to find healthy food. When we arrived in that historic city lined with brick streets and horse-drawn carriages, the only thing on my mind was breakfast, lunch, and dinner.

It's safe to say I spent about sixty percent of the trip looking up restaurants and menus. My dying phone battery would probably agree with that assessment. While walking the streets carved by palm trees and century-old churches, my eyes remained fixed on Yelp and Tripadvisor.

I stumbled across a vegan, clean eating restaurant for brunch. *Success.* Yet, my heart and nose drifted to the smells of southern classics like fried catfish and biscuits and gravy that came out of local establishments. Childhood memories of my Aunt Sue's home cooking from Kentucky flooded my head, but the voice within told me a bowl of chia seed pudding with fresh fruit would have to do. The vegan joint represented an opportunity to try something new, even if it wasn't covered in butter and gravy.

The people working and dining at the vegan restaurant glowed with vitamins like the Instagram influencers I idolized. Everybody seemed so perfect, so healthy, so pure. The clean white walls, house plants, and juice bar enamored me. I strived to be just like the workers and patrons.

Luckily, my craving for biscuits vanished with each spoonful of that colorful chia pudding. It was a heavenly marriage of creamy yogurt and crunchy coconut bits mixed with fresh berries.

This is it. This is the pinnacle of healthiness. I am devoting my life to clean eating.

The next day dumped more fuel on the raging fire for eating perfection. Matt and I planned a day trip to Asheville, North Carolina. This last-minute addition meant I needed to recalculate my breakfast plans. I identified a vegan restaurant nestled in the pines of the Blue

Ridge Mountains. While I wasn't vegan, this cafe seemed advanced for its time in the western Carolinas. I hoped for a repeat of the day before.

"Looks pretty healthy," I assured Matt, who was also looking for a lighter option to close out the trip.

Matt decided to try their vegan "soysauge" and I was willing to take the plunge with him. It was our first endeavor into meat substitutes.

The patty came out and looked just like the pork ones I grew up on. My tastebuds sang in joyful chorus with the first bite. The sage shone through. The flavor exceeded that of real sausage. The texture fooled my mouth into believing this was the real thing. Another seed was planted when I devoured that patty. Vegetarianism tasted mighty fine that Saturday morning.

Later, Matt and I made a surprise trip down to Clemson University. My heart beat a little faster being back in a college town. Matt found a little ice cream shop yet again. This man's love of ice cream cannot be denied. I was at ease when we walked in and found it doubled as a coffee shop.

Perfect, I'll just get a decaf to numb my hunger and resist temptation.

However, the smell of the fresh waffle cones and the growing line of college kids trumped the bitter coffee grounds. I wanted ice cream so bad. After all, we were on vacation, right?

Look at all those college kids devouring their icy delights. Then they get to go act their age and be real college students. Ugh.

I sat in a cushy leather chair, judging each student as they reached for their cones. Jealousy raged, disappointment rumbled, and the constant reminder of my inadequacies ruled the evening. Nonetheless, I forced a smile and joked with Matt even though I just wanted to get to the room and sleep.

CHAPTER 19

PANCAKED

During one of my investigations into clean eating, I stumbled across a Keto website. Their colorful chart ranked various fruits and vegetables in terms of carbohydrate and sugar count. It became another bookmarked website for quick reference.

Sweet corn, a summer staple for a boy from the Midwest, found itself on the dark side of the chart, as did melon, pineapples and pears. Welcome to food jail, my sugar bomb friends.

After the successful meals in South Carolina, we introduced more plant-based proteins into the diet. Soon, my beloved salmon swam into the pond of limited quantities. The amount of fat in each filet caused my heart to flutter. I spent hours each day researching the healthiest diets. At work, at home, it didn't matter. I combed the Internet for the key to eternal youth and longevity. Alternative flours, cauliflower everything, and protein shakes became my new best friends.

Pizza, a former lover, was now on the forbidden list with the exception of the time I found a cauliflower crust recipe on one of my health food blogs. Matt, the honorable soldier he was, agreed to make the crust to resurrect pizza night. He spent two hours in the kitchen cooking the cauliflower, then straining it, and cooking it again, until the once-firm florets finally resembled a mushy pile of playdough.

The apartment smelled nothing like a pizzeria. A sour odor drifted from the oven to the couch where I sat nervously awaiting the results of the experiment. The finished product looked like a pizza, but the pale crust came with a bitter aftertaste.

"Wow, this tastes really good," I said, smiling. I tried to fool myself and Matt into believing it was worth all the effort he put into it.

Matt responded with a look of disappointment and a monotone, "Yeah, uh-huh."

Weekend meals looked like weekday meals; the variety was gone. Matt was also dieting now to get in shape for the wedding. But his diet was much more relaxed than mine. He still incorporated treats, and he wanted to have special date nights at the mouth-watering Tex-Mex establishments which dot the Houston landscape.

As my strained relationship with food hopped the elevator to the next floor, my actions started putting pressure on the relationship. Matt loves pancakes, and he always cherished weekend mornings. They were his opportunity to flip up a couple flapjacks. His constant pleas for pancakes often meant one of my many excuses.

"Oh, I already ate."

"Um, not today."

"We're going to have a big lunch."

And so on.

"Do you not like my pancakes?" Matt growled one morning from the kitchen.

"No, I'm just not in the mood for pancakes today, that's all," I said.

I never meant to hurt his feelings.

Just watch what you say so he doesn't get suspicious.

I really did love his pancakes. I often suggested alternative flours, protein powder, or ingredients that could help ease my anxiety, but the pancakes turned out tasting like burnt grass every time.

"We should just stick with my recipe," Matt grumbled after each failed attempt. Deep down, I knew he was right, but the thought of just one bite left me paralyzed.

As summer turned to fall, which actually doesn't exist in Houston, I gave in.

"Why don't you make your pancakes tomorrow?" I asked one afternoon. I had devised a plan.

That next morning, when the sweet aroma of batter and cinnamon filled the apartment, I rested easy. I had eaten my chia pudding and overnight oats before Matt woke up, making sure to quickly wash the utensils and cover my tracks before Matt got out of bed.

When Matt set the fresh plate of pancakes on our patio table that morning, he drizzled his pancakes in sticky brown syrup. I decided to go dry.

The pressure of my fork revealed the perfect balance of fluff and chew. My mind raced in a million different directions as my boney hand closed in on my lips. I chewed, relishing and hating the taste, before I grabbed my white paper napkin. A quick swipe to the face was my magic trick. I spit the mushy pancake into that napkin while swallowing nothing. I glanced over at my soon-to-be-husband.

Phew, he didn't catch me. It worked.

I did this several more times as the ball of mushy batter grew in my palm. I tossed the evidence in the garbage can the first chance I could get and piled things on top of it for added insurance.

⁓

A few weeks out from the wedding, the mirror revealed a skinny Jason. However, thousands of dollars' worth of personal training yielded little in terms of muscle growth. My arms were still the twigs my friends often joked about. Protein-heavy meals, protein shakes, and countless hours in the gym produced a jiggly wimp.

What is wrong with my body?

Maybe I don't have what it takes to be a real man, to have muscle and be athletic.

At the same time, I bragged every time a friend or family member remarked on how skinny I was. Skinnier meant more attention and, most of all, better health.

CHAPTER 20

THE DESOLATE MAN

My dad's side of the family hails from south-central Kentucky. Dad was the only one who moved away from the Bluegrass State's rolling fields. Our trips "back home" were the highlights of my childhood. The eight-hour drive to Kentucky couldn't go fast enough. I loved seeing my aunts, uncles, cousins, and grandma.

We always spent the week between Christmas and New Year's at Grandma's house nestled on the outskirts of bucolic Glasgow, Kentucky. In between crocheting blankets, she'd be in the kitchen whipping up country ham, creamed corn, and buttery biscuits. She loved to make food. My grandma was known around the county for her fried apple pies. I can still taste that creamy, spicy filling wrapped in a flaky buttery crust.

I looked forward to playing with my cousins. Since my siblings were so much older, it was nice to have peers I could relate to. My cousin Shane and I played video games for hours, while his mom, my Aunt Sue, catered to our every need. "Y'all want ice cream sundaes? How about some cake?"

I always cherished the early mornings at Uncle Russell's car shop. The smell of oil and grease made me feel like a man, even if I wasn't more than knee high to a grasshopper. While Dad and Uncle Russell talked, I imagined I was on a NASCAR pit crew. My imagination ran wild in the safety of that small shop in the country.

Glasgow differed from the exploding suburbs of Chicago. They even had Sonic. Oh, and a Dairy Queen with food. I always returned to school after a trip to Kentucky eager to tell my friends about my southern roots. As a kid, I didn't see the social and religious divisions. Instead, I saw the kind loving people that always had my back.

After my dad passed, I grew even closer with the Wood family. They were my closest remaining connection to Dad. The feeling was mutual. I loved hearing stories about their childhood and what my dad was like as a kid. I'd spend weeks at a time in Kentucky during the summer just soaking up the slower way of life with people I admired. My stomach ached by the time the trip was over. Weeks of non-stop laughter and my aunt's homemade cooking took their toll.

Things changed after Mom's death. My sister Lori had reached out to my Kentucky kin with concerns about my partying and life choices. While she may have been doing so out of worry for my well-being, it drove a wedge between my aunt and me. Alcohol is the devil to most of the Wood family. Heck, Glasgow was in a dry county up until 2016. Just the thought that I could enjoy a party lifestyle turned my aunt away from me. Lori was right; I was hiding things from them, but only for my own protection.

What if they find out I'm liberal or, even worse, gay?!

I'll lose them, too.

Losing them felt like losing the last part of my dad that remained. The frequency of my trips down I-65 dwindled. My fingers didn't dial up the 270-area code as much. I kept them at arm's length to protect them from my "wild" city life. Self-exile seemed better than abandonment.

I approached my wedding guest list with cautious optimism. Most of my dad's family did not know about my sexuality. Some knew Matt as a friend and roommate. Only a very select few knew we were together. This burdened me for years because I wanted them to know how amazing he was. Similarly, I wanted Matt to see how much these people and Kentucky meant to me. Sending them a Save The Date with their beloved nephew or cousin kissing another guy would probably not go over too well, but it was a risk I had to take. I was done living in disguise. More importantly, I wanted them there on my big day. With Mom and Dad gone, these folks had to be there in the front row, supporting me and loving me.

Anxiety bubbled when I dropped the Save The Dates in the mailbox.

Here goes nothing.

The postcards slammed against the metal bottom of the mail slot as my heart slammed against my rib cage. Weeks passed with no response from Kentucky.

"Did your parents say anything about the wedding?" I asked my cousin Shane via text.

"No, I haven't talked with them about it. They haven't said a word."

I tried to reassure myself. I figured they just needed the formal invite to RSVP. If they weren't supportive of my homosexuality, they probably would have already said something.

The wedding invites went out in late June. Responses trickled in, but the silence from the land of bluegrass was deafening

Was there an issue with the post office?

With the deadline approaching, I started calling some of the Wood folk. They never answered or followed up on my voicemails. Another piece of my heart broke with each ring of the telephone. I soon realized none of my aunts and uncles would be coming to the wedding, minus my uncle's ex-wife, who remained close through it all. God bless my Aunt Bev! The most damaging part was the fact they didn't even acknowledge it. Not even a "no" or an "I'm disappointed in you." None of that—just radio silence from my dad's kin.

CHAPTER 21

WEDDED WORRIES

A month before the wedding, my sister texted me, offering to throw a small wedding shower for us back in Illinois. I showed Matt the text message, shocked.

"That's very nice of her to offer," Matt said with cautious optimism. "Do you think it will be awkward?"

The fond memories of big holiday get-togethers with my siblings lingered in my mind, even if they felt tainted following the estate battle. My siblings and I had started talking to each other again more recently as we realized we all grieved and hurt in different ways after Mom died. A part of me knew that they thought they were doing the right thing by objecting to my partying and life decisions. But I still held resentment for the way things turned out. So I kept them at arm's length with full defenses up. I guess you could say I practiced social distancing before it was a thing.

Matt and I accepted the invite. And before we knew it, we found ourselves on the front porch of my sister's home. My stomach felt like it was playing a game of Twister, and Matt looked like a soldier going off to battle.

The door opened to several rounds of, "Oh wow, you're so skinny," and "You need to eat more." As usual, I took it all with mixed feelings of pride and frustration.

All four of my siblings were there that afternoon with my nieces and nephews, some of whom I hadn't seen in ten years. Matt was soon laughing it up with his newly formed "out-law" posse, which consisted of him and my two sisters-in-law. They considered themselves brave people for voluntarily marrying into this crazy family.

Matt and I ate our plant-based sausages, to the murmurs of how gross they looked. "How can you eat that stuff?" one sibling asked. I shoved it down with pride. "It's better for you than red meat. That causes cancer and I have to be careful with my colon polyps."

My heart and stomach felt full in the setting sun, yet I could not escape the haunting memories.

Why did it have to turn out like this? Was this all my fault?

I chugged another glass of red wine as Lori pulled out old photo albums. "Look Matt, here is Jason in middle school," she giggled, pointing to a picture of "Fat Jason" complete with oversized glasses and bowling trophy. Sure, I was embarrassed, but isn't that what big sisters are supposed to do when you bring home your better half?

"Okay, we should get going soon," I whispered to Matt when Lori retreated upstairs to grab more photos. What I really wanted to say was, "I'm sick of everyone commenting about how skinny I am, and I'm hurting because I feel like I'm the reason this family fell apart."

~

September meant wedding time. I couldn't wait to finally say I do to Matt. However, fear lurked in my mind.

What will I do after the wedding? Will I return to eating badly on the weekends? Are carbs suddenly okay again? Will I get fat and unhealthy as a result?

I planned every minute detail of the wedding, yet food remained the wild card. We were getting married back home in Chicago and then going on a week-long mini-moon to Michigan. This meant more temptation to cheat on my strict diet. It also represented the end of my shield from worried friends and family. Their remarks at how skinny I was, or my new strict diet, could easily be defended by saying it was for the wedding. That excuse would soon be invalid.

Our maids-of-honor coordinated the rehearsal dinner with much input from yours truly. We planned an intimate event with just the wedding party and several close friends at a local pizza joint. They reserved a small back area off the bar for our party. I made sure not to eat too much pizza that night and focused on loading up my plate with salad.

Tomorrow is the big day. Your chance to shine.

I found it difficult to focus on the conversation with non-stop food police radio traffic in my head.

Load up on salad. Eat lots of greens. You can do this. Roger that.

Towards the end of the meal, our maids-of-honor Kate and Sophia mentioned they had a surprise for us.

Oh no, surprises are never good.

"We know there will be cake at the wedding tomorrow, but what kind of friends would we be if we didn't celebrate with this one first?" Sophia asked, beaming with joy as she set the infamous Portillo's chocolate cake in front of Matt and me. The whole table turned its attention to the decadent layers of moist chocolate cake slathered in rich, creamy frosting.

It looked like a work of art. But the cake cast a shadow on my mind.

"Oh my God! This looks incredible, thank you!" Matt exclaimed. He wasted no time grabbing the knife to dive in.

"Wow, you guys are awesome! Thank you," I said, my lips curling into a forced smile. But my heart sank.

Okay, well you have to eat some of this cake. You're so lucky to have these people in your life. Show them you're grateful.

"Just a tiny slice for me," I said as Sophia started dishing out pieces. "I've got to fit in that wedding suit tomorrow after all." Laughing nervously, I wondered if my suit wouldn't fit. And what if the sugar was feeding undetected tumors?

"Why don't we share a slice?" I asked Matt when he gave me a piece much too large for my liking. "It will be good practice for tomorrow, and I'm already stuffed."

To my relief, Matt agreed. At that point I figured I could just eat a couple bites to appease everyone and get back to the hotel. But the entire table seemed fixated on watching Matt and me eat the cake. I usually love being the center of attention, but at this point I was hoping for a meteor to strike the parking lot—anything to take the attention off my gluttonous act.

"Here, you two take the rest of the cake with you." Kate said. I looked down to see three quarters of the beast remaining. Even though I wanted to throw it in the garbage, I knew my friends had spent a lot of money on it. I struggled with wanting to appreciate their gift, and stick to my diet plan. I went with keeping the cake, with no intention of eating it.

"Sure, we've got a fridge in our suite," I said. "This will taste great later."

~

I worked out like normal on my wedding day, hit up Starbucks for my safe "oatmeal," and dug into my safe stash of hard-boiled eggs and fruits in the hotel room. Friends offered to take me out for breakfast, but I turned to my long list of excuses to prevent the guilt that would ensue from a meal out. I already knew the rest of the day would be a free-for-all.

My best man Joe and I hit up a bar for lunch. I planned this outing for weeks, so I entered the bar prepared. We watched some college football before suiting up ourselves. Go Hawks! The menu revealed many enticing options, including the chicken wings Joe ordered. But I resisted and went with Salmon pasta, the dish I identified weeks earlier during my restaurant reconnaissance. I declined the sauce and only ate a couple strands of angel hair. *Protein, protein, protein.*

I had made it through the last meal before the wedding.

The ceremony and reception went off without a hitch. We dealt with cold temperatures, a blustery wind, and occasional mist, but it was still a dream come true. My planning paid off.

Matt looked incredible in his suit. I still look at pictures of him in the navy blue suit and can't believe he was my groom. I even felt handsome that day. Sure, I had to settle for a custom suit thanks to my calves, but I still felt like a character out of Downton Abbey. For the first time in years, I found confidence in myself.

This confidence couldn't help me overcome dessert, however. An assortment of mini cupcakes dotted the dessert table. I knew I would have to eat cake.

Two days in a row, really?! But who doesn't eat cake on their wedding day?

In classic wedding style, Matt and I interlocked our arms and shoved a mini cupcake in each other's mouths. Friends and family laughed, as did we, while capturing the moment with their iPhones.

Guilt still tickled my mind when we saw the feast back at the hotel after-party. The buffet of pizza, sliders, and tater tots looked to die for, but I wasn't willing to die for it. I nibbled on a corner slice of pizza and a few tots. Even though it was my wedding day, and the big event was over, I found it difficult to treat myself.

The food fest continued the following morning with a doughnut and champagne brunch in our suite to say farewell to our guests. Eight dozen coconut, blueberry cake, and sugar-raised donuts, ordered from an old-school doughnut shop my father and I frequented often, were displayed on a large wooden board. When the sweet aroma hit my nose, I felt like I was back at the doughnut shop with him. But this time, doughnuts were "bad," and I was bad for eating two of them.

With two dozen doughnuts left over and that Portillo's chocolate cake screaming at me in the mini-fridge, I insisted that each guest take some treats home with them. No one hesitated, thanking me for the generosity. I smiled back at my friends, but only because I could get all the desserts from the wedding out of my sight.

It was then that I realized my wedding diet was now my full-time diet.

CHAPTER 22

MILE HIGH EXPECTATIONS

The coming months signaled the end of our Texas days. Our jobs and desires led us to the Mile High City of Denver, Colorado. This meant that I needed to find a new gym, new safe restaurants, and even grocery stores.

Mountain life is welcoming, calming, and adventurous. In Denver, you can grab the best beer of your life at one of the dozens of breweries or be up in the mountains in no time skiing or hiking. The city feels like an oasis from the stresses of life; however, I could not escape the stress of my eating rituals. Surrounded by half-empty moving boxes and disassembled furniture, I went to work identifying healthy eating options near our new apartment. Turns out, it's pretty darn easy. Coloradans are active and take care of themselves. The local dining establishments reflect that lifestyle.

First and foremost, I established where the closest Chipotle was to adhere to my strict burrito bowl lunch rules. Then I made it a point to research the healthiest options in town for weekend breakfasts and dinners. Rather than fully explore Denver's dining scene with an open palate, I often promoted only the places the Internet or I deemed healthy enough.

Within weeks of our arrival, I crafted lies and exaggerations about my life to fit in. I told fellow Hawkeye fans at the local alumni bar that I also went to Iowa for college. Sometimes I'd go as far as stealing a friend's life story about growing up in Iowa to further the fib. It felt easier to play a persona because I was embarrassed by who I really was.

It wasn't long until I made a group of friends. Happy hours and spontaneous get-togethers for the game were a thing again. This development blurred my focus on my strict eating regimen. Alcohol tended to do that. Suddenly, a beer and slice of pizza on a Tuesday night were not off-limits. I started indulging in hops, greasy bar food, and good times.

After the strictness of the wedding diet, my thirst for freedom took hold again. I started getting belligerent when I drank. The once fun-loving, happy drunk now revealed a dark side. Matt and I fought more. I would often say things that hurt him; things I didn't mean. I just wanted someone else to feel the pain I felt inside.

The scariest thing of all is that I didn't remember a lot of these occurrences. I used to pride myself that I could down a twelve-pack and remember everything the next day. Now my memory felt like a redacted document.

Matt didn't seem to share the same excitement about our new home. He can't drink due to an alcohol intolerance, so he rarely joined me on my trips to the bar. Rather, he stayed at home or went shopping while I painted the town.

Each morning after drinking, I promised myself I wouldn't drink that day. But by noon, I found myself making drinking plans with friends all over again. I could feel the excitement building as we discussed where we would go, and what time we'd meet up—excitement I felt robbed of when I had missed out on college nights out. College seemed to finally be happening, just fifteen years late. However, just like college, this experience came with a heavy cost.

The wedding pictures on the wall felt like they were from another lifetime. Just four months after our nuptials, I wasn't just pushing Matt away. I was pushing myself away.

CHAPTER 23

HIT THE CURB

We'll all remember where we were when the COVID-19 pandemic started. Matt and I happened to be in DC for my regularly scheduled colonoscopy. Watching the news in our hotel room, Coronavirus seemed like another one of those diseases with a big media bark and measly bite. But before we knew it, March Madness and the St. Patrick's Day Parade were canceled. Bars and restaurants started closing, and the governor eventually closed the entire state. Matt and I couldn't even go to work.

This was no false alarm. We were entering a life-changing and unprecedented time.

Thankfully, Matt and I made it back to Denver early that Saturday morning. I went out with my friend one last time before the shutdown. We celebrated with green jello shot after jello shot and enough beers to make an Irishman blush. After hours of endless booze, I stumbled to pick up pizza for dinner. The chain of events that followed assaulted my mind for months.

With so few dining options still open due to the shutdown, I stumbled to a go-to pizza joint. This was the hot spot, evident by the line of people I found wrapped around the building.

The next thing I knew, my face met asphalt. In my drunkenness, I had missed the curb and wiped out—a belly flop right there in the street. I heard several in the line erupt with laughter. I hopped to my feet, tried to play it off, and ran around the corner. Tears flooded my eyes. The shame and embarrassment from the high school locker room flashed before my mind. The cool guy persona I thought drinking gave me vanished with a thud. I was that fat kid in gym class again, the kid who had to wear husky jeans, the family's disappointment, the gay outcast.

"Where's dinner? You were supposed to get pizza," Matt snarled as I stumbled in the door. I slurred my way through an explanation of what had just happened to me. I was a belligerent mess of tears.

Lacking any sympathy for my drunk ass, Matt stormed off to the bedroom. We went to bed that night clothed in tension, matching the changing world around us.

Once Matt woke up, I apologized for the night before and vowed to never let it happen again. I'm happy to say I stuck true to my word. The next three months ushered in sobriety. Granted, this was made easier now that bars and restaurants were closed. I took immense pride in my ability to stop drinking. I figured that since we were stuck at home, I could spend this time fixing myself.

～

Early in the pandemic, Matt jokingly referred to me as the social distancing police. I'm a rule follower, not just with my food, but in every aspect of life. I started getting confrontational with people who didn't follow local rules and guidance.

One day I referred to a young lady as a "fucking bitch" when she jogged past us at a close distance without a mask. It reached the point where I couldn't leave the apartment without returning in a fit of rage. My disdain for society grew.

Maskless folk and anti-social distancers infuriated me. I viewed them as the obstacle to returning to normal. In other words, they became the puppet master. I had no control over the situation, and I needed control.

I developed a phobia of people. I shifted my morning walks to before sunrise to avoid others. I stopped going to the grocery store and ordered everything for delivery. I even switched up the dog's potty schedule to avoid neighbors in our building's elevator. Just a few months ago, we were in a new city with endless opportunities ahead. Now, we were confined to a 700-square-foot apartment.

When the offices closed, I saw my responsibilities as an office coordinator reduced to nothing. I woke up every morning with no meaning or purpose. It was either sit on the couch and watch daytime television, or use this time to become a healthier, happier person.

The overachiever within grew frustrated with the lack of productivity and took drastic action. With everything else in the world spiraling out of control, I returned to one thing that produced the feeling of productivity and accomplishments: my diet and weight. With alcohol already cut out, I figured this was the time to regain my health.

My first step was vegetarianism. I eliminated meats from my diet, justifying the decision based on animal cruelty and personal health. But deep down, I recalled how red meats always came up on the colon cancer risk factor list. I thought about all the glowing, "pure and clean" people I saw at the vegan breakfast spot back in Charleston and desired to achieve their level of health.

I also reimplemented rules for carbohydrate limitation. This made my new vegetarian lifestyle tricky. A large portion of my previous routine consisted of grilled chicken. Now, it was replaced with chickpeas. So long Double Chicken Chipotle burrito bowls! Welcome to the bad list.

My workouts didn't feel as accomplished from home. I walked for almost an hour every morning and then returned home for another hour of cardio or weight training. Exercise even replaced watching sports as my new favorite hobby. And rather than plan events and happy hours at work, I spent most of my day planning the healthiest menu I could find. The list of good foods shrunk with every Google search or Instagram click. The list of bad foods exploded.

Matt and I joined a virtual baking club. I loved spending time with him in the kitchen, but I hated the thought of eating the fruits—or should I say carbs and sugar?—of our labor. To reduce any suspicion around my eating habits, I returned to the old pancake-in-a-napkin technique. I'd take a bite and then spit the baked good into my napkin and bury the evidence at the bottom of the trash can.

My caloric intake reached a new low, but that was never my intent. I was just eating the foods I saw as "clean." The scale continued to drop lower and lower, which felt like a bonus.

"This is the best I've ever felt," I bragged to my friends. "This clean eating and abstinence from alcohol is exactly what the doctor ordered."

No one seemed concerned. In fact, my friends were in awe of my determination.

The thought of an eating disorder never crossed my mind. I still ate daily and wasn't concerned about appearance or body image at the time. After all, in the middle of a pandemic, it's not like you're being seen.

The long-burning flame within reached the wildfire stage. My deep self-loathing and the unresolved issues from my parents' deaths popped and crackled. The reduced responsibilities at work reminded me of my unaccomplished life. My new healthy lifestyle now defined who I was and became my full-time job.

CHAPTER 24

FEELING THE EFFECTS

The shutdown continued through the summer of 2020. Stuck at home, I volunteered to assist in any way I could. The news was bleak with riots, political divisiveness, and a rising death toll. I needed to help.

Without an office to manage, my job became obsolete. Thankfully, my employer kept me on, but I had nothing to do. The events I planned to throw were all canceled. Only a couple of months into my dream job, it was put on indefinite hold. I needed something, anything, to do to still feel like a productive individual.

In June, I assumed the role of a volunteer contact tracer. I expected to make dozens of calls a day. Instead, we had a minimal workload. Most people we connected with weren't interested in completing the interview.

Very few foods remained on the good list by this time. Every day felt like rinse and repeat; same breakfast, same lunch, and same ingredients in a different combination for dinner. The scale continued to give me glowing performance reviews. I dipped to the lowest weight of my adult life. Pain and weakness started to creep in, tempering the internal joy of my regular meetings with the dictator scale.

That summer was among one of the hottest in Denver's history. We experienced a record number of days above ninety degrees. Wildfires raged across the state. A fire raged within, too, but it wasn't enough to keep me warm. In fact, I spent most of the summer shivering and bundled up on the couch, draped in a hoodie and blanket. The indoor thermostat often cracked eighty degrees. My only reprieve was in the late afternoon when the sun shone through the living room windows. I wore a winter coat during my morning walks, even as the air temperature hovered in the sixties and seventies.

Must be this thin mountain air.

Veins poked through my skin like rows of dirt in a freshly planted field. The images of vein-bulging bodybuilders on social media reassured me that these changes were normal and a sign of total health. My hair started falling out in the shower. It looked brittle like straws of hay. My once-a-week nail trim graduated to every other week.

Perhaps my nails are growing stronger because my blood is just pumped full of nutrients.

Sitting down became a literal pain in the ass. I could only sit for ten minutes at a time before fidgeting around. Pillows didn't seem to help. Working out also became painful. My elbows dug into the hard floor during planks, causing an episode of bursitis. Russian twists felt like some sort of torture tactic. My hip bones plowed right through the foam of our extra-thick yoga mat into the hardwood floor. Workouts left me exhausted if I could even get through them without feeling dizzy. I figured it was a sign that I was really pushing myself now.

At one point, Matt voiced concerns over the lack of intimacy in our relationship.

"Do you not find me attractive?" he asked one evening as we settled on the couch for dinner one night. "Why won't you touch me?"

"No, you're so handsome. I love you!" I said, feeling shame rise within. "I just don't have much of a sex drive right now."

I was also embarrassed by the way I looked. I wanted to look like the fit bros online, not the frail alien-like creature I was morphing into.

Already lacking confidence as a male, this was the cherry on top.

CHAPTER 25

INDEPENDENCE DAY

After months stuck at home, Matt and I jumped at the opportunity to escape for a few days to Wyoming around the Fourth of July. A long weekend and a decline in COVID cases provided the window we needed to make our great escape.

Fort Collins was our first stop. The bustling downtown area is bordered by rocky foothills and gorgeous hiking trails. We started the trip off with a hike around the sparkling waters of Horsetooth Reservoir. Then we visited several of Fort Collins' breweries for a couple of cold beers to cool off from the summer heat. Matt and I were having a great time until a fit of anger consumed me while strolling Colorado State University's shaded grounds.

My eye doctor had failed to provide a copy of my contact lens prescription before closing for the long holiday weekend. Irate, I called them and left a nasty voicemail in the middle of our tour around campus. Several profanity-ladened threats later, I hung up. I shook with anger and rage. Matt remained silent, knowing not to poke the bear. I rebounded after this episode and managed to enjoy the rest of the day. Looking back, I feel like this was a precursor to the events that followed.

I managed to find some level of control in my life when I spent the car ride up to Wyoming researching restaurants. I was relieved to find several suitable lunch options in Laramie, but when we arrived, we found most were closed for the holiday. My anxiety levels rose to level orange. Next stop, code red.

"Well, drive down this street. Maybe we'll find something there," I sighed, exasperated. After nearly an hour, we saw a local pizza joint that was open with outdoor seating. In other words, they checked two out of three boxes. I tried desperately to find a healthier alternative but to no avail. Hanger was imminent, so I bit the bullet. Pizza it was.

In my attempt to get the healthiest option, I ordered a small margherita pizza with light cheese.

"Who eats pizza without cheese?" Matt would often remark whenever I ordered pizza.

"When I worked at Domino's, lots of people did it because of intolerance," I would reply, justifying my dairy-free decisions. Granted, I didn't suffer from any dairy intolerances.

When the server brought out our pizzas, they looked average at best. As a Chicago boy, I know a good pizza when I see one. But I was pleased by the deep red tomato sauce shining through the gaping holes of the limited mozzarella pools on top.

I muddled my way through half the pizza until I reached what I guessed to be fullness. I still don't know if I was full, or if my mind just told me I was. Either way, I felt like I had just gained twenty pounds. My stomach pushed at my waistband, while my shirt suddenly felt tighter around the chest. The pizza was subpar, totally not worth the calories, carbs, and fats.

Matt didn't seem all that thrilled with his pizza, either. We put our napkins down and hopped in the car for the hour-long journey to Cheyenne. But even in the car, with each passing mile marker, all I could think about was the pizza I was sure was clogging my arteries.

For dinner, I identified a place in downtown Cheyenne where I could eat the hummus platter for an appetizer. But I had one condition: I needed to replace the pita with raw vegetables. This was common, as Matt would enjoy the pita while I loved my fresh veggies.

"Sorry, we don't have any fresh vegetables we can give you," the waiter explained upon our request. The waiter's words ripped through me like dynamite. My deer-in-the-headlight eyes met with Matt's.

"Um . . . we'll need a few more minutes," Matt replied.

When the waiter walked away, I snapped.

"I just want to leave. I'm not going to eat anything. I just want to go to bed," I said, my voice shaking and on the verge of tears. "I hate this city, this place, everything!"

I felt heavy from pizza, frustrated with the endless search for healthy options, and now irritated at a restaurant with no fresh vegetables.

Matt's eyes tensed up. "Please calm down, Jason. We'll come up with something else to eat," he said in his deep soothing voice. I, however, was past the point of no return.

"I just want to go home, back to Denver. I'm done," I said.

"What's wrong, Jason?" Matt asked. "I'm worried about you. You need to eat more, and it's just a pita. It won't hurt you."

How could I put my fear of that flat, round, carbohydrate monster into words? And how would Matt possibly understand? But what Matt said next changed my life.

"Do you think this has something to do with everything you've been through with the death of your parents and losing your family?" he asked. "Like some sort of PTSD?"

I froze. This was the first time I'd heard Matt acknowledge my past like that. In fact, this was the first time anyone had said it. I don't remember what I said back to him, but I knew this changed something in me. I needed someone to say this out loud for me to feel like it was a problem worthy of help.

Through my tears, I grabbed the pita and ate several bites. It tasted great. Matt acknowledged this big moment with an encouraging smile. But while I enjoyed the pita, I knew, sitting there under the cloudy skies of Cheyenne, that I was sick. I was not in control like I thought. This—whatever it was—was bigger than me, and I needed help.

When we returned to the motel, Matt promised we would leave first thing in the morning. I was eager to leave that night but agreed with Matt that we should get some sleep.

I spent most of the night shivering on the cold tile of the bathroom floor to be near a faucet since running water comforted me. The hot steam enveloped my body like a protective fog. My stomach ached, growling for food after the measly plate of pita and hummus.

I lay there, grappling with the thought of getting help, and feeling like a field mouse under the eyes of a hawk.

CHAPTER 26

HELP ME, PLEASE

I figured I didn't have an eating disorder. I believed that my situation did not match the eating disorders I learned about in school. But I knew I had some issues to work through, so I scheduled a virtual appointment to meet with my primary care physician. Settling down on the couch for my virtual visit with the doctor, I felt anxiety cut through every corner of my insides.

What will he think of me? Am I crazy? Is there really anything wrong with me, or am I just being dramatic?

When my doctor appeared on screen, I let everything out. I confessed that I was unable to treat myself to foods on my "bad" list because they stoked overwhelming fear and guilt within. I talked about how long that list of forbidden items was growing. It was getting to the point that even some fruits and vegetables were no longer allowed. I let him know I desired complete control over every aspect of my life, including my diet, amid the chaos of the pandemic. I mentioned my recent fits of rage and anger, including the pita incident in Cheyenne.

With each word, I felt better. Revealing my secret to someone other than Matt felt liberating. Scary but liberating. My doctor remarked that I showed signs of anxiety, obsessive-compulsive disorder, and an eating disorder. He referred to my condition as an unspecified eating disorder. "I'll have to add this to the patient portal as 'Eating Disorder – Bulimia/Other' since that is the closest option to your situation."

I found that odd terminology since I had never once thrown up any food, nor did I really binge. The label didn't match my condition, leaving room for doubt. Did I really have an eating disorder?

"Okay, what are the next steps?" I asked.

My doctor prescribed an SSRI medication for me and advised that I seek counseling. I asked him for referrals.

"Take a look online," he suggested. "Mental health resources are limited right now. It's best to just look around and see who accepts your insurance and what fits your needs."

If I had pain in my stomach, you would give me the name of a gastroenterologist to contact, I thought. *Or if I had a weird spot on my skin, you would give me the name of a dermatologist.*

At this point, I thought I had already taken the biggest step forward by admitting I needed help. However, I didn't know what that help would look like. Apparently, neither did my doctor.

I figured it couldn't be that hard to find a therapist to treat my problems. I would just do what I always did: turn to Google. However, when I typed in "male therapist for eating disorders, OCD and anxiety," I mostly found local eating disorder clinics for in-patient care. Their websites were painted with images of women who spoke about their battles with anorexia and bulimia. None of this was relatable to me.

Perhaps I'm just a guy who has some weird relationship with food.

Already at my lowest point mentally, physically, and emotionally, I gave up my search.

Maybe I'm just not fixable. Maybe I'm sentenced to this hell I've been living in for so long. And who knows, this unspecified eating disorder thing sounds made up, so maybe I'm not really that sick.

I resumed my search after a couple of days. I decided to focus on my anxiety and OCD first. They seemed like easier topics to find a therapist for. I later learned that this was the right decision for my situation. I stumbled across that revelation on my own without any medical guidance. I was lucky.

I sent out approximately twenty messages to prospective therapists referring to my unhealthy relationship with food. Note the terminology here. I still didn't believe I had an actual eating disorder.

The majority resulted in the following responses:

"We're currently not accepting new patients."

"We can schedule you for a consultation in 3 months."

"We're unable to help you with regards to your specific conditions."

Some of the therapists never even responded. I feared I would be broken for the rest of my life. Then like an oasis amid scorched earth, I received a message from a counselor named Sean. In his email, he explained his belief in helping clients find their voice and draw upon their inner strengths. This appealed to me because I felt I had lost my voice and my identity. I didn't feel strong at anything other than controlling my food intake.

Sean and I met a few days later for a virtual consultation. He looked like your typical Colorado dude: average Joe meets outdoor adventurer, and not much older than me. I felt an immediate connection.

Stumbling over my words, I told Sean that I suffered from disordered eating, anxiety, and OCD. Sean's smile and occasional nods as

I recounted the events of my childhood and adolescence reassured me that I was in the right place.

"Now, Jason, I must admit I haven't worked with many clients who are dealing with eating disorders. But I would love the opportunity to work with you through this hurt and anxiety."

Maybe I am valid and worthy to get help.

Sean and I scheduled a time to meet the following week for our first full session. The prospect of working with Sean reminded me of going to haunted houses as a kid. I was excited and scared witless at the same time. I didn't know what to expect.

The inner skeptic wondered if it would even work.

CHAPTER 27

MINDFULNESS MATTERS

During our first session, I provided Sean with a high-level overview of my life: the weight loss, the deaths of my parents, and the family turmoil that ensued. I talked about my need for control and my obsessive planning nature. I told him I enjoyed those aspects of my current diet.

I also shared with him my recent outbursts and growing frustration at the world. Sean suggested I start engaging in mindfulness techniques. During the call, we spent five minutes tensing up and then relaxing portions of the body, starting from the toes and working to the head while focusing on breathing. He recommended I try this technique the next time I felt things slipping out of control. I remained doubtful this would work, but the part of me that always needed to excel in school took over.

Jason, trust the process because he is the expert.

Over the course of the next week, I engaged in this mindful technique on several occasions.

Close your eyes, curl your toes, feel the pressure, then release.

I felt my anxious and obsessive thoughts subside with each repetition.

Because the apartment Matt and I were in was located on the fourth floor, we made several trips a day on the elevator to take the pups out. A few residents regularly ignored the signs posted requiring masks and allowing one party at a time on the elevator.

My entire body would tense up each time the elevator opened. The ignorance of some residents used to send me into a fit of rage, which usually involved me returning to our apartment with several choice words and a knot in my neck. However, I noticed my new breathing techniques seemed to quell that anxiety and anger I felt while riding the elevator with a maskless individual. It seemed Sean was on to something.

I took immense pride and satisfaction in planning weekend excursions. During the shutdown, I put together theme nights at home with activities to keep our minds off the world outside. These activities helped make up for my inability to plan work events. They also made me feel like a contributing member of the household.

However, I had planned too much on one hot summer afternoon soon after starting therapy. Matt and I had already walked nearly two miles for brunch that morning in the blazing mountain sun, and now I was dragging him to a brewery.

"Why aren't you talking much?" I asked at our picnic table next to a grilled cheese food truck. "Did I do something to upset you? What's wrong?"

"Nothing. I'm fine, just tired," Matt said. He avoided looking at me, telling me he wanted to be left alone.

What did I do? What did I fail at now?

I thought I planned a fun time.

I finished off my drink before we made the quiet walk back to our apartment.

At my next session, Sean and I dissected the experience. He helped me understand that things like this can happen. Matt was tired, that's all. I didn't do anything wrong. There was no need to beat myself up over things that didn't go according to my high expectations. This was my first breakthrough.

I saved several inspirational quotes I found online to my phone. They served as extinguishers to my anxiety and anger and eventually found their way into my recovery journal. My favorite one was "Never let a bad situation bring out the worst in you. Be strong and choose to be positive." I shared my findings with Sean at the next session, who remarked on my initiative. Just like school, I was learning and improving. It was satisfying to my inner perfectionist and overachiever.

I renewed my vow to trust Sean and the process. From there on out, I opened up about the grief I went through with my parents' deaths, and the insecurities with everything that happened in the family afterward. We unearthed pain and memories I didn't know were there.

Just weeks after I started therapy Matt and I decided to participate in a virtual 10k near the end of July.

"You know, I was thinking we should complete the event at Garden of the Gods," I said. For someone who previously equated nature with snakes and injuries, this was a big change for me, and Matt noticed.

"Wow, that's a great idea!" Matt said. "What made you pick that?"

I told Matt that it would be worth trying something different, and that I was ready to try new things and break out of my comfort zone. He couldn't object to that.

Two weeks later, Matt and I arrived at the park just after sunrise. The scenery seemed like something out of a National Geographic special. Red-orange rocks spiked towards the blue heavens from the luscious greenery below. Within moments on our hike, we stumbled upon a herd of elk in the morning mist. Goosebumps ran up my arm and neck.

I couldn't believe this was at my doorstep the entire time. My therapy sessions opened my life up to adventure. Next stop, climbing one of Colorado's famous 14ers.

Sean assigned homework at the end of each session. He always laughed when I came the next week ready to show off my work.

"Most of my clients don't even do these," he said smiling. "You go above and beyond."

Sean told me it meant a lot to him as a counselor to work with someone who engaged in the process. The straight-A Jason beamed with pride over the progress I was making. The strengths I didn't realize I had were making themselves clear, and my determination and commitment to learning broke through the storm clouds of my past shortcomings.

Three assignments will stick with me for the rest of my life. While too personal to post on the fridge, I keep them saved on my computer as reminders.

The first one was a letter to my sister Lori, a letter that will never be sent. In it, I express how much I loved her when I was younger. We were best friends. She was my big sister and my idol; however, things changed when mom passed away.

I wrote about the conversation we had in the car the night before mom died when Lori called me a disappointment; the words that broke me for years. I blamed Lori for selling my dad's legacy, for judging me and driving a wedge between my family and me. I expressed how I felt robbed. Emotions that had lurked beneath the surface for fifteen years flooded out into that word document.

Yet, I closed with a thank you. When you're younger it may feel like adults are out to get you. When I looked back on the experiences with my sister, I began to understand her perspective. And as hurt as I was, I know the way she handled everything came from a place of grief and love.

I read the letter to Sean, and later, to Matt. As the last word left my lips, a tumultuous chapter of my life ended. I no longer hated myself for the way things turned out. I no longer resented Lori. I realized our relationship would never be close, but I finally let go of the anger and pain.

Sean sat in awe of the letter. He remarked on my writing talents, praising my ability to share my story.

I loved writing in school. Essays, poems, narratives, you name it, I loved writing about it. My favorite college courses were the ones that involved the most writing.

I recalled writing a poem after my dad's death. My Uncle Eugene saved it in a dresser drawer for years and showed it to me during one of my last trips to Kentucky. It reminded me of how much I had missed my dad, and how much I missed writing.

Reflecting on all of this, I realized a strength that had been there all along: writing my truth.

Sean proposed a new writing assignment, much to my excitement. I had peeled back twenty years of grief and pain, and Sean recognized that I never had a chance to grieve the loss of my mom. A week after her funeral, I started a full-time job at Domino's Pizza just trying to survive financially. A month later, I started my turbulent chapter of constant relocation.

So Sean asked me to write a eulogy for her.

Tears poured down my face with each keystroke. Some were happy tears as I reminisced on her over-the-top holidays with presents taking up half the living room and enough cookies to feed the entire town. And there were sad tears, too. I wanted to hold her hand one more time and twist her wedding rings around those wrinkly, soft knuckles like I did when I was kid. In the letter, I introduced my mom to Matt, and to who I was as an adult.

Sean listened as I read my mom's eulogy. A moment passed after I finished. And then, in a shaky voice, he said, "Wow. Thank you."

The third writing assignment from Sean focused on writing out my story. He thought this would be a good tool for sharing my battle with friends. Boy, was he right!

After I typed up the initial draft of my story, I read it back to myself. Like Stephen King suggests, we must first tell ourselves the story before we can tell others. As I read through paragraph after paragraph of my life's journey, I realized something. I was simply doing the best I could given the circumstances. Reading my story from a third-party, objective point of view allowed me to start forgiving myself for past failures and shortcomings. Above all, it enabled me to start loving myself again.

Those assignments helped me realize that I was always doing the best I could. This allowed for self-forgiveness and self-compassion. The past no longer haunts me. I can open the family picture album and feel joy again. Those memories are no longer tarnished by the fallout from my mom's passing.

Free from my past, Matt and I began planning the future. Next up, that overdue honeymoon to Italy.

Speaking of planning, I now limit my daily to-do lists to three items or less. I no longer have to overachieve or set unrealistically high expectations.

I am doing the best I can. I am enough.

Empathy and patience have also infiltrated my social interactions. Recognizing my struggles has enabled me to see that many other people have their own battles. Additionally, I learned to expect the unexpected. My first test came at a quaint French Bistro in downtown Aspen several months after starting therapy. The server had made a mistake with my order, and Matt was the first to see it.

"How did they not know there was bacon in that quiche?" he grumbled. "I'll talk to the manager. This is ridiculous."

I took a deep breath. "You know what? It's fine. Why don't you finish up your lunch and then I'll grab some food at the brewery around the corner. No biggie."

Matt did a double take, stunned. "Wait, who are you? What did you do with hot-headed Jason?"

I laughed and reminded him that I am now Jason 2.0.

CHAPTER 28

TRUST

My newfound strength and confidence from working with Sean finally enabled me to take the next step: address the disordered eating. However, the search for a dietitian once again yielded a whole lot of nothing. Clinics with teen girls discussing their anorexia didn't seem like the right fit for me.

Sports nutritionists seemed a little more suitable since I wanted to build muscle and stay healthy. I scheduled an initial consultation with one, but I found she was not prepared to work with someone fighting an eating disorder. She suggested that I follow her standard meal plan and drink several protein shakes. From her perspective it seemed as if my eating disorder was only about the food. I needed a dietitian who understood the voices and urges telling me not to eat, an individual who could help me see the good in food again.

After several days of searching, I stumbled across a registered dietitian's website that appealed to me. "Intuitive Eating" was posted across the webpage. I had never heard of the concept before, but after a quick scan, I learned that intuitive eating promotes a healthy relationship with food by making the individual an expert in listening to their body's hunger queues. It's the opposite of dieting. Intuitive eaters listen to their bodies and eat what they want. This sounded like an opportunity to break free of my constant obsession with food.

I loved everything this dietitian, Kassandra, spoke about. However, I noticed no mention of eating disorders. I worried she might not be able, or willing, to help a guy like me. Like Sean, Kassandra hadn't worked with many individuals in my situation. But after our initial consultation, she was willing to take on the case.

"We'll conduct metabolic measurements and genetic testing to see how your body responds to macro and micronutrients," she said, voice alive with optimism and confidence.

My mind exploded at the thought of freedom from the chains of dieting. If I could learn about my body from an almost academic approach, then maybe I could start to forgive some of the forbidden foods. Unfortunately, that joy was doused when I received Kassandra's follow up email. I learned this program was not covered by insurance and came with a hefty price tag.

I flung myself on the bed in tears. I didn't want to put that financial strain on Matt and me for some nondescript eating disorder. Matt, like he always does, reassured me that I was worth it.

"The most important thing is helping you get better," he said.

The next day, I enrolled in the nutrition program with Kassandra.

At my initial visit, Kassandra and I decided to get rid of my scale to prevent me from obsessing over the numbers. Matt wasted no time evicting that sucker from the house. Kassandra and I also decided that I would only weigh in every other week during my office visit.

Kassandra had one of those high-tech scales that measures body fat, lean muscle mass, bone, and water. It also breaks it down by limb and torso for a complete look at each area of the body. The printout from my first weigh-in had more "unders" on it than Tiger Woods' scorecard. Every section of my body measured underweight in both fat and muscle mass.

I couldn't help but think I was still in a good place. After all, isn't it better to be under than over? But then I learned that I was at high risk for a sudden cardiac event. My pulse was slowing, and my blood pressure registered well below normal. I read about several athletes who felt fine and then dropped dead in the blink of an eye. The strain of their intense fitness routines and diets proved too much for their vital organs.

Okay, maybe this is more serious than I thought.

My doctor confirmed that I needed to get my weight up. I was in dangerous territory. With the pandemic still raging, I feared that one bout with COVID could decimate my ill-prepared body.

Kassandra crafted a meal plan with my preferences in mind. She made sure to consider that I wanted to remain vegetarian for ethical reasons. While I may have been initially seduced by the health benefits of a plant-based diet, I was now better educated on the environmental benefits of vegetarianism. And if I still wanted a chicken nugget now and then, it was fine. The only food rule now was that there were none.

Kassandra asked me what foods I liked. Of course, I only listed off the foods on my "good" list. While she took my preferences into account, she devised a plan to match my needs.

The first week's meal plan scared me because there were foods like honey, peanut butter, and bread—foods I still thought would kill me. But I knew that I had to trust the process. The countless tests Kassandra performed reassured me that she knew what was best for my body.

The next week felt like a nonstop battle in my head. First, I couldn't believe how much I was expected to eat. I had to include snacks? I was used to just three meals a day. Snacks seemed like something gluttons ate.

I made my own loaf of bread that week chock-full of whole wheat flour, oats, and seeds. This made my return to bread a little easier. If I was going to eat bread, I was going to be damn sure it would be the healthiest recipe I could find.

The voice inside remained steadfast.

Should you really be eating that?

What if this bread increases your cancer risk?

Are you sure that's the right serving size?

I decided I had to write a message on our letter board to fight back, reading "DEFUND THE FOOD POLICE."

Two weeks later, I entered Kassandra's office. I was nervous and a bit hopeful that the scale would show my hard work. Kicking my flip-flops to the floor, I stepped up on the silver platform across from her desk. The green arrows instructed me to grab the handles and squeeze. A few seconds later, the digital numbers that appeared deflated my balloon of confidence.

I was down three pounds.

How could this happen?

Maybe this isn't the perfect fit for me after all.

I failed, again.

I put the handles down and turned to Kassandra who looked deep into the light radiating from her computer screen. She read the numbers off the monitor and reassured me this could happen. "Your body has been deprived of nutrients for so long that your metabolism is probably out of whack. We'll up your caloric goals and see if that does the trick."

I hung my head in shame as I got back in my car, still grasping onto the printout of my results. I sat in the parking lot, looking over every metric for a sign of hope.

How am I going to tell Matt? He'll be so disappointed. And I've wasted all our money.

Then something dawned on me. I ate all those additional calories, the so-called "bad" foods like a peanut butter sandwich, and I didn't gain any weight. Plus, I had more energy again. Okay, there it was. My glimmer of hope appeared: maybe these foods weren't so bad after all. I returned home cautiously optimistic about my future.

"How did it go?" Matt asked.

"I lost three pounds, I'm sorry."

Matt's face lost all excitement. "What happened?"

"Well, Kassandra said this is common, I guess. We're going to up my caloric goals. But hey, look at it like this. Who cares what the scale says? I'm feeling better and eating more of those 'bad' foods again. That's got to count for something, right?"

Who was this person speaking? Was this the same Jason who feared carbs just a few weeks earlier? Those words signaled change beyond anything a scale could measure.

"Yeah, that's a good point," Matt agreed. "Keep up the good work. I know you can do this!"

Sean also applauded this newfound perspective. The divorce from Mr. Scale seemed to be going well. I was ready to trust the process again.

The increased caloric goals still seemed daunting at first. How was I supposed to climb Everest when I was still learning to conquer a molehill? The voices in my head wanted to use the new goals as ceilings to avoid. The "less is more" mindset proved hard to break. After all, this was a habit I developed during my Weight Watchers days in high school. But this was not a number to stay under. This was a number to hit, a target to aim at. I had to embrace the challenge in front of me.

My strengths were always there, just sometimes used for the wrong purposes. My overachiever tendencies pushed me to succeed. Instead of searching for healthy restaurants and analyzing menus, I redirected my search for new recipes focused on healthy, wholesome eating. I realized foods I had deemed "bad" actually had benefits. Honey and maple syrup satisfied my sweet tooth while filling me up with crucial minerals. Salt was a flavor booster, not just a heart attack waiting to happen. I expanded my culinary tastes and fell in love with new cuisines like Indian, Thai, and Ethiopian. Yes, the voices still screamed at me, but I needed to gain weight to regain health and happiness.

The subsequent weigh-ins revealed modest gains, making the overachiever in me frustrated. B's were nice. But I wanted A's. No, wait, A-pluses! Does it come as any surprise that my favorite emoji is the red "*100?*"

Meanwhile, Sean and I addressed how I was often my own worst enemy. He talked about the Buddhist concept of the two darts. The first dart represents an unavoidable event in life that inflicts pain, like my mom's death. The second dart is self-inflicted when we criticize our response to the first dart, much like the pain and self-hatred I carried for so long.

Yes, first darts are unavoidable no matter how hard we try to protect ourselves. Life happens. But we have control over the second darts—our reaction to the traumatizing event—and subsequent response. In my case, the second dart wedged in my soul for years. It twisted every time I felt like a disappointment in the wake of my mom's death. It pushed deeper each time I suppressed my pain and put on an act.

My awareness and mindfulness of these second darts have now enabled me to maintain inner peace even in the face of pain or disappointment. I guess Sean was onto something when he taught me that mindfulness technique during our first session.

This concept carried over to my slow weight gain. The numbers on the scale meant nothing. My accomplishments were much more than some digits on an electronic device. With every meal, I was getting better regardless of what my weight revealed.

The walls of my comfort zone were crumbling. I stopped using the "good" versus "bad" debate to judge food. Even better, I stopped using it to define myself. I started to learn self-compassion in the face of pain or disappointment. My recovery could not be measured by numbers alone.

CHAPTER 29

NEWFOUND FREEDOM

Before recovery, I didn't spend much time in the kitchen. In fact, I hated it. The few times I cooked or baked, I usually ended up with blackened French toast complete with a ruined pan, bland shrimp stir fry, or a liquidy pineapple upside-down cake. Who knew that skim milk was not a good substitute for sour cream?

Recovery, however, ignited my inner Gordon Ramsay. I began bookmarking new recipes and organizing them in numerous sub-folders, of course. I could eat healthy while still eating foods I once viewed as the bad guy. Rice and pasta were welcomed back to the pantry. Their friends cereal, real milk, and peanut butter also joined the party.

"Is that what I think it is?" Matt asked, eying a store-bought loaf of bread I had just brought in.

I grinned. "Yes, sir!"

"You haven't allowed that in the house for years. I'm so proud of you!"

"Jason 2.0, thank you," I laughed.

As the food rules loosened, the kitchen didn't seem like such a bad place.

Trips to the grocery store became less stressful. If they didn't have my organic bananas, I allowed conventional produce back into my shopping cart. Ordering in from restaurants still stoked the voices within, but I worked on telling them to hush.

A few weeks into recovery, Matt and I went out for breakfast to celebrate. We picked a local cafe with an outdoor patio. I refrained from looking at the menu all week, causing my heart to race as we took our seats at the sunny sidewalk table. I opened the menu to a world of freedom. This was a breakfast for two: Matt and me. Orthorexia was not invited.

"You know, I think I'm going to get the biscuits and gravy," I said.

"Oh wow! Look at you! No egg whites or yogurt parfaits?" Matt quipped.

The waitress brought out a heaping plate of flaky biscuits smothered in a shiny pool vegetarian sausage gravy. I felt like that young boy at McDonald's again. This was my new version of a Happy Meal.

"This looks incredible. I can't believe I'm doing this," I said, smiling.

"I'm so proud of you, Jason. Eat and enjoy."

My fork plowed through the biscuits until nothing remained but a few crumbs. My stomach felt full, not fat. My mind was full of joy, not guilt.

~

It's safe to say that our first year of marriage did not unfold the way we thought it would. Who could have seen a pandemic stopping the world in its tracks? This did not stop us from celebrating our first anniversary in September 2020. Matt and I rented a rustic log cabin just outside Aspen. Mountains of fall colors waved in a new beginning. We had a lot more to celebrate than just our marriage.

Previous trips ignited anxiety over food and dining options. If the level of anxiety around those trips was a wave, it would be at tsunami level. This time felt more like a lazy river. Meals no longer required intense planning. We ordered pizza, sushi, and doughnuts without fear or regret. I found myself waking up each morning with a clear head and anticipation of a fun day of adventure ahead.

There were still some ripples along the way, including one last pancake-in-the-napkin experience. Matt and I had stopped off in Vail for a quick lunch. After eating doughnuts that morning for breakfast, my inner critic suggested a smaller lunch. I obliged.

Then Matt asked me to try a bite of his meal. To avoid looking like a failure at recovery, I agreed. Old habits die hard. I chewed a couple times and then lifted the napkin to my mouth. I turned my head and spit out the food. While I thought I had been sly, Matt saw. I sensed the tension as we climbed back into the car. A few miles down the road, Matt spoke up.

"Can I ask you something weird? Did you spit out the bread earlier? There was mushed up food in the napkin I threw out."

I confessed and told him about my previous actions with this technique. I feared that I ruined our trip and disappointed Matt. To my surprise, the confrontation strengthened me. Matt and I held an open conversation about why I felt the need to spit the food out. We had broken down another barrier to recovery. Recovery is a process, not a pass/fail test. It's okay to have a bad moment because those thoughts don't vanish overnight. There was nothing to hide.

I could share my thoughts and concerns without judgment.

CHAPTER 30

THE MISSING PIECE

The structure of learning new information, applying it to real-life situations, and then testing it out always appealed to me. I decided it was time to take a real-life course in recovery from anxiety, OCD, and eating disorders. So I ordered several books on overcoming anxiety and OCD in addition to eating disorder recovery. This could be my secret weapon in recovery. It turned out to be one of the best decisions of my life.

I'm an early riser, usually awake by 5 a.m. After my morning workout, I plopped down in the comfy chair in the corner of our dining room. While sipping my decaf, I read for about an hour. This newfound hobby paid rich dividends as the books supplemented my work with Kassandra and Sean. I learned about techniques to overcome the anxious thoughts in my head.

The first piece on eating disorders was authored by dietitian and eating disorder warrior Libby Parker titled *Permission to Eat.* Her story opened my eyes to the eating disorder world, a world I avoided for so long because I felt it didn't apply to my situation. But now I realized that maybe this wasn't just some weird relationship.

True to its title, this book granted me permission to eat. Libby's words tore the rule book from inside my mind and tossed it in a burning fire. I began to accept that I was battling an eating disorder, not disordered eating. At my next session with Sean, I said the term "eating disorder" casually in conversation.

"Wait, stop there," he said. "Do you know what you just said?"

I paused, thinking. Now that I admitted that this was an eating disorder, there was no going back. Sean and I celebrated the moment, knowing that this was a turning point.

A few days later, I found myself immersed in another book called *Goodbye Ed, Hello Me* by eating disorder warrior and speaker Jenni Schaefer. In it, I stumbled across a new term, "orthorexia." With the curious mind I have, you know exactly what I did. If you said Google, then you've been paying attention.

I typed in the term, and BAM! You would have thought the Iowa Hawkeyes just won the national championship in our dining room. I placed the laptop down on the table and sat in a state of stunned disbelief. This was it. That is what I had been fighting.

I do have an eating disorder, and it has an identity. I'm justified in needing help. It's so much more than just some weird relationship with food.

I was ready to rip out another dart that had been lodged in my mind for years. Shadowed in the darkness of an early October morning, I could suddenly see everything so clearly. I hadn't been this speechless since Matt proposed to me.

How had I never even heard of this disorder before?

It took every bit of energy to not scream it from the rooftop, but I knew Matt needed his beauty sleep. Instead, I admired the sunrise, which looked extra beautiful that morning. The darkness finally came to an end.

The next couple of hours were spent researching orthorexia. I read about Dr. Steven Bratman, who first coined the phrase in the mid-90s to describe his patients who had an unhealthy obsession or fixation with healthy eating. Every article shed further light on the thief that stole so much from me. My personality traits and OCD, as well as my insecurities about weight in childhood and dieting in adolescence, made me a ticking time bomb for this disorder. The matches were lit long ago and then turbulent times in my life added the fuel needed to spark an eating disorder that burned through every aspect of my life.

Some people in the eating disorder and mental health field refrain from labels. I see their point that it may trigger an individual or worsen the condition. But for me, this was a declaration of independence. Once I knew my enemy, I could defeat it.

Sitting with my notebook out and numerous studies on the screen, I probably looked like a mad scientist when Matt made his way down the stairs into the dining room.

"Orthorexia—have you ever heard of it?" I asked, jumping out of my seat. Still half-asleep, Matt mumbled and shook his head.

"That's what I have," I declared, abruptly ending his transition from slumber to life. I rambled on about my new discovery over the buzz of Matt's electric toothbrush and the rattling of the tea kettle.

Like a detective with a lead in a cold case after twenty years, I spent the next few days ordering books on orthorexia and searching for resources online. As I gathered more information, I wondered how I had not come across the word before. Why didn't anyone mention it? Especially my doctor? Why hadn't my support team or Internet searches revealed this term? How could I have been sick with something and controlled by it for years without even knowing it had a name? Why were social media influencers and food bloggers pushing the clean eating rhetoric without also warning it can become too much?

Orthorexia is not recognized as a formal eating disorder diagnosis. While studies and interest in the topic are growing, there are no official diagnostic criteria for the illness. That's why it's often grouped in with the phrase "unspecified eating disorder." I can't stand that label. It's like selecting "other" on a questionnaire. It underestimates the power orthorexia holds over its victims.

I will admit I was skeptical about the scale of my toxic relationship with food for some time. But now that I know what orthorexia is, I can see the damage it causes.

CHAPTER 31

THE VULNERABLE SURVIVOR

I can't put my finger on the moment when a healthy diet morphed into a life-threatening eating disorder. My goal was to live longer and maintain a healthy lifestyle. I thought I was doing the right thing by tracking every calorie and macronutrient. I believed working out several times a day, seven days a week, was the ticket to perfect health. I trusted that healthy, clean eating would give me the control I needed to be satisfied with the person I was.

In reality, It was the eating disorder that was calling the shots.

As I progress through recovery, I can see several factors that played a role in the development of my orthorexia, from the bullies as a kid and my extreme dieting in high school, to the stigmas and stereotypes around men's mental health. On top of that, there was the steady influence from social media and diet culture telling me I was doing the right thing.

The seeds were planted long before the pandemic; it just happened to be the catalyst that saved my life. Unfortunately, there are many more individuals out there like me.

If I had learned about this obsession with healthy eating in school, I wouldn't have been lured into this dungeon. If just one of my friends, my husband, or even my doctor had heard of this term, then my journey to recovery may have begun much earlier.

When I first sought help in July 2020, I asked Matt to refrain from telling anyone else. There was no way I could let the people who were closest to me in on this dirty secret. Would they still like me? Would I still be fun to hang out with? Would they think of me as a liar and a fraud? As a drama king? Or worse, a weakling?

I voiced my concerns to Sean during our regular weekly session. He reminded me of my strengths and asked, "What do you have to offer your friends? What kind of friend do you want to be?"

I realized that I wanted to be an empathetic, compassionate friend after all the years that I had been an inmate trapped behind the bars of strict food rules. Orthorexia forced me to skip out on social events. And even when I was present for my friends, my mind often drifted into what I would eat next, how I could avoid "bad" foods, and what I ate the day before.

While my friends had seen bits and pieces of the real Jason over the years, many of them had never seen the Jason I was becoming in recovery. I was ready to be the authentic, true Jason I always was. But this scared me, too.

My best friend Kate had witnessed my tough life experiences, from facing homelessness to battling my opinionated family. After I explained my latest obstacle, orthorexia, and apologized for being so distant, she responded in a sympathetic tone.

"You were in survival mode, dude."

∼

One night, Matt and I watched a Brene Brown special on vulnerability. This talk perfectly supplemented Sean's encouraging words about how being vulnerable is a sign of strength.

Vulnerability is defined as the quality or state of being exposed to the possibility of being attacked or harmed, either physically or emotionally. All along, I was the one doing the attacking and harming myself by not allowing myself to be vulnerable and share my struggles.

I finally found the courage to be vulnerable with friends and share my eating disorder battles with them. My closet of masks and personas was tossed to the curb. I was no longer starring as another character in this production. It was time for my true cameo appearance.

Embracing vulnerability is a major step outside of the comfort zone. My eating disorder and anxiety thrived in my comfort zone, but now that I have stepped out, I'm the one who is thriving.

Take, for instance, my new favorite hobby, rock climbing. Old Jason would have been terrified. The challenge of climbing a wall and getting to the top is much like the challenge of eating six meals a day in recovery. There are some places where I feel stuck and don't know how to proceed, but I just keep going. It may get uncomfortable at times but that's when the growth occurs. That's when I reach the top, but I'm damn sure enjoying the process along the way.

Now I am sharing my story with the world because I never know who needs to hear it. The response has been overwhelming. Some friends and co-workers have since disclosed their own unhealthy relationships with food and eating disorders with me. Our level of connection has grown through this embrace of vulnerability.

My friend Katie sends me regular text messages reminding me of her love and respect for what I've been able to overcome. I also notice I receive a lot more messages from my friends just checking to see how I am doing. Our friendships have evolved beyond just funny quotes or sports talk.

It gets even better. Now when I meet strangers, I get to be me. It makes social interaction a hell of a lot easier. The stress of hiding behind a curtain of lies and inner pain is no longer there.

My race is far from over. The intrusive thoughts are still there, but they've gone from screams to whispers. I remind myself of the statement on the inside cover of my recovery journal: "TRUST the process, EMBRACE the process, and eventually ENJOY the process."

I don't know what "recovered" looks like. I don't even know if that state exists. But what I do know is that I'm beating orthorexia and my inner demons every day. A recent setback reminded me of this.

While on vacation for Matt's birthday, he wanted ice cream for dessert. Already feeling a little uneasy because of the change in my daily routines, my anxiety heightened as we approached the ice cream parlor. I walked through the doors to that seductive smell of waffle cones before getting slapped in the face with the calorie counts on the menu board. My mind immediately went to that *"sugar will kill you and you will get fat, you failure"* place. I panicked and was unable to order anything that evening.

However, rather than beat myself up about my setback, I loved myself for trying and promised I could do better next time. The next morning, Matt and I headed out for breakfast. I opened the menu to once again be greeted by numbers galore.

"Oh no, do you want me to read the menu to you?" Matt asked.

"No, I've got this. Orthorexia won last night. I'll be damned if it wins again today."

I ordered my pancakes complete with fruit topping and whipped cream. I even asked for a side of eggs. It tasted like sweet victory.

When I wake up each morning and look out at the mountains surrounding Denver, I'm reminded of how I've conquered my own mountains. And in those moments of reflection, I am back in my parents' bed, talking with my dad. I tell my dad about my fears, my insecurities, my dreams, and my life.

In recovery, I recognized that those late-night conversations with Dad growing up exemplified what a man of the house should do. He embraced vulnerability and held space for me. He encouraged open and honest conversation. It's ironic to think I spent so many years doing the exact opposite to appear manly.

With this book, I am keeping my promise to Dad and living my life as the man of the house. However, this man is taking out the garbage of stereotypes and stigmas.

Men battle eating disorders. Men battle mental illness. Men hurt, too.

Trust me, I know a guy!

ACKNOWLEDGMENTS

First and foremost, thank you to my rock, my refuge, my best friend. Matt, you came into my life at one of the darkest times and instantly brought light. Now, more than a decade later we continue to climb past obstacles and celebrate victories together. That evening in Cheyenne when you raised your concerns about my unresolved pain and eating habits saved my life. Your love and courage at that moment empowered me to start my road to healing. I'll never be able to fully explain how much your love means to me. Look at that, you left me speechless! But I will say that this journey, the blog, and this book have all been made possible by your love and support. We've got this!

I also want to thank my best friends who love me for me and have always been there when I needed them. Kate and Joe, thank you for opening your doors when I needed a place to stay or shower. Kelly, thank you for being my best friend since Kindergarten. You are the one I can always go to reminisce about mom's crazy antics and you're always good for a laugh when I need it. Katie, thank you for your words of encouragement. You've always reminded me that I am enough, even if I didn't always see it. And to all of my friends who have stood by my side through the good times and the bad, I thank you! Thank you for the holiday dinners with your families and the memories that will last a lifetime. It really is true, friends are our chosen family, and what a beautiful family I have.

Through my blog and advocacy work, I've been able to grow this family. Matt B., you inspire me every day with your will and determination to overcome obstacles. Your poetry and writing have had a profound impact on me. I'm so grateful to Molly and Diane for helping to connect us. I look forward to continuing our Friday chats for years to come and can't wait to get to a White Out Game with you!

Then there is the one and only Paula Quatromoni. Paula, I never dreamed of the impact a simple email could have. Thank you for your heartfelt response and encouragement to not just start sharing my story, but to write this book. The work you are doing is saving lives. Thank you for being an ally in the fight against stigmas and stereotypes. Your students and this world are lucky to have you!

And without Paula, I may have never met Rachael Steil who guided me every step of the way through writing, editing and publishing this book. Rachael, thank you from the bottom of my heart for sharing your own story of survival in *Running in Silence*. You helped me find my voice and will forever be a mentor and friend.

Also, thank you to all of the individuals who helped out as beta readers. Some of you have already been mentioned, but your feedback was critical in ensuring this story leaves an impact on those who need to hear it. You've made me a stronger writer and storyteller, but more importantly, you are helping to change lives.

Dr. Jason Negata, thank you for your research and advocacy of men and eating disorders. You are challenging the status quo and changing the narrative around men and mental health. I am overwhelmed with gratitude for your contribution to this book.

And to the readers and supporters of Orthorexia Bites, I am grateful for every single interaction we share. The Internet can be a rough place at times, but you've shown me the power of connection and community. You are the mental health movement this world needs! Please know you continually inspire and empower me.

I would also like to thank all of the individuals who have invited me on their podcasts or platforms to share my story. I often say there is so much power in storytelling. This applies both to the audience and the individual sharing their story. You all have enabled me to continue healing while helping others overcome their own battles. Keep up the great work!

I must take a few moments to extend my heartfelt gratitude to my support team of Sean and Kassandra. I'll never forget how scared I was the first time I met both of you. I was embarrassed by my life. I was broken. I had my doubts treatment would even work, but the warmth and support you showed me quickly inspired me to trust the process. Together, we've been able to address obstacles I didn't even know existed. Thanks to you, I am now able to share this story and hopefully help others. I'm ready to pay it forward!

Lastly, I have to take a few moments to thank two individuals who are no longer with us. My parents, Darlene and William Gordon Wood. Memories of the good times we shared bring me comfort on tough days. Your individual stories of overcoming challenges strengthen my resolve in the face of adversity. Your love for the little things reminds me of how truly blessed I am. Our time was cut short here on this Earth, but your lessons and legacy live on within me. I felt you by my side as I wrote this book and know that you will always be a part of my life. For that, I am forever grateful.

CONTACT THE AUTHOR

Jason Wood manages the blog Orthorexia Bites, contributes to various podcasts and mental health projects, and speaks about his battle with orthorexia and mental illness to audiences around the world.

You can find out more at OrthorexiaBites.com and follow on social media here:

Twitter: @OrthorexiaB
Instagram: @OrthorexiaBites